ADVANCE PRAISE FOR *Birth Matters*

"In her captivating down-to-earth, common-sense style, Ina May opens our eyes to the normalcy and trustworthiness of our birthing bodies. This book provides a beacon in the darkness of today's maternity care."

—Penny Simkin, author of *The Birth Partner: A Complete Guide to Childbirth for Dads, Doulas and All Other Labor Companions*

"In her wonderful book, Ina May Gaskin manages to be both sane and inspiring. Crucially, she calls for feminists to reconcile women's power with the powerful experience of birth."

—Jennifer Baumgardner, author of *Manifesta, Look Both Ways,* and *Abortion & Life*

"In *Birth Matters*, Ina May shares with readers the wisdom she has gained from her *four decades* of midwifery experience, and her wide-ranging study of interconnected women's health issues ... She honors women's capacities for giving birth autonomously, unmedicated, and strongly believing in their own powers."

—Jane Pincus, co-founder of Our Bodies, Ourselves

"Ms. Gaskin is a bright light shining into a dark chasm of forgetting ... I believe we should do well to hold Gaskin's writings up among the great philosophical contributions to our time."

—Ani DiFranco, from the foreword

BIRTH MATTERS

a midwife's manifesta

INA MAY GASKIN

FOREWORD BY ANI DIFRANCO

Seven Stories Press
NEW YORK

A Seven Stories Press First Edition

Seven Stories Press
140 Watts Street
New York, NY 10013
www.sevenstories.com

College professors may order examination copies of Seven Stories Press titles for a free six-month trial period. To order, visit http://www.sevenstories.com/textbook or send a fax on school letterhead to (212) 226-1411.

Book design by Jon Gilbert

Library of Congress Cataloging-in-Publication Data

Gaskin, Ina May.
 Birth matters : how what we don't know about nature, bodies, and surgery can hurt us / Ina May Gaskin. -- Seven Stories Press 1st ed.
    p. ; cm.
Includes bibliographical references.
ISBN 978-1-58322-927-9 (pbk.)
  1. Natural childbirth. 2. Labor (Obstetrics) 3. Midwifery. I. Title.
 [DNLM: 1. Natural Childbirth. 2. Delivery, Obstetric. 3. Feminism. 4. Midwifery. WQ 152]
 RG661.G375 2011
 618.4'5--dc22

                                        2011001677

Printed in the United States

9 8 7 6 5 4 3 2

This book is dedicated to the heroic men and women who have put their own careers on the line to provide the best possible care for women and babies.

Contents

Foreword

My parents' marriage exploded when I was very young, and like the survivor of a sunken ship, I found myself drifting off into the adult world as a teenager. At sixteen I had several jobs, my own apartment, and some strong survival skills that hinged on a sense of personal invincibility. Having sewed confidence and capableness into my identity, I pursued life as an emancipated minor without fear. I was rewarded with a wonderful career in music, a grand adventure that led me from stage to stage around the globe and further emboldened my independent self-image. At the age of thirty-six, when I was pregnant and looking forward to giving birth, there was a voice inside of me that said childbirth would be easy for me—that I would get through it as I had gotten through everything in life, without pause. I chose to give birth in my home with a very low-key midwife, adverse as I was to the fear mongering that I believe leads many women into hospitals and into the hands of controlling doctors. I stand behind my choice, and believe I was right about all of it except for one thing: childbirth would not be easy for me. It would be a dark and at times fearful journey that led me to unforeseen places including a crisis of identity.

Late one night, three weeks before my "due date," my water broke and so I stayed up 'til dawn scribbling excitedly in my journal while my partner slept soundly upstairs. In the morning I went to the hospital to confirm that this weird discharge was indeed amniotic fluid and was strongly advised to check myself in and submit to chemical induction because of "risk of infection." Believing more in the wisdom of Mother Nature than the wisdom of doctors, I went home. Over the next several days my labor ebbed and flowed but in the middle of the third sleepless night, I realized I was headed towards a brick wall of exhaustion and began instinctively marching up and down my stairs to propel my nonlinear labor forward. This worked and I progressed to the pushing stage but being so weak with sleep deprivation I pushed for five hours unsuccessfully. My contractions flared dimmer and dimmer and somewhere in the background I heard my midwife say, "I think we may need to go to the hospital." I was given a cup of tea with a lot of honey and some much-needed advice: "Try to stop pushing and rest through as many contractions as you can. See if the sugar helps revive you." I lay there in a dark sea of crisis and delirium until, clear as day, I felt the sugar enter my bloodstream. I waited until I felt the full power of that cup of tea and then with the words "we may need to go to the hospital" ringing in my ears, I summoned my lover and my midwives back into my sphere. "OK now," I said and pushed until by Goddess my daughter's head came out.

If I had it to do again, I would invite more of an atmosphere of accompaniment and camaraderie around me. I would call upon confident women to put their arms around me and rock me and clap hands and growl and make me laugh down the fear. Though it was the most painful thing I've ever experienced, I do not regret giving birth naturally.

One of the downfalls of our excessively comfortable society is the idea that pain is a bad thing to be avoided at all costs. We have built great pharmaceutical empires bent on masking, subduing, and eradicating pain, even emotional pain, from our lives. We are taught to view pain as an enemy, not a teacher. But pain is the right hand of growth and transformation. Pain is in the history of all human wisdom. The pains associated with menstruation and childbirth (even the emotional pain) are the price of having agency with the bloody, pulsing, volcanic divinity of creation, and they lie at the core of feminine wisdom. The literal experience of

my body is your body
your blood is my blood

holds great insight into the way of things. A self-possessed woman in childbirth can be a powerful teacher for all (including herself) on the temporality, humility, and connectedness of life. What if the medical establishment that purports to be saving women from the specter of pain and danger is instead ejecting them from the seat of their power?

I have many friends now who have given birth, most of them in hospitals with a myriad of interventions, and a truly shocking number of them by cesarean section. Young, healthy, and strong women. It confuses me that I, an educated, privileged woman in twenty-first century America, am surrounded by women who think they need saving and, because they are denied the opportunity to know otherwise, may believe it forevermore. They look at me with wide eyes and say, "I couldn't have done what you did," and my heart breaks as I think quietly, "Yes, you could have! In fact, I bet you could have done better!" How could all these otherwise empowered young women go so unquestioningly into the role of damsel in distress when it comes time to have their children? How were they convinced that they "couldn't do it"?

Ms. Gaskin is a bright light shining into a dark chasm of forgetting. With this new book she once again illuminates from her vast life experience not just practical and reliable pregnancy and birth information, but also an opportunity for us to remember the power and the purpose of childbirth. I believe with her that the ripple effects of turning this most profound moment of female empowerment into its opposite are immeasurable. Pregnancy and childbirth are meant to be a time in women's lives when they bond with other women and all of womanhood (if they haven't already), and come into a new sense of themselves and their capabilities. What happens when eons of feminine wisdom are buried under the shifting sands of important men and their machines? What happens when women lose control over the fundamental processes of their lives? What would happen if instead, women were encouraged to believe in themselves, their bodies, and their instincts? What if there were an atmosphere of respect and deference to mothers, in which women were empowered to access their inner strength and wisdom, as well as the wisdom of eons of women who have come before them? What if society acknowledged all the ways in which Birth Matters?

Interestingly, in this book we hear Gaskin's account of trying to interface with the feminist hegemony along the way. One that all too often attempts to blur the lines between male and female and focus on how well women can succeed within patriarchal frameworks if given half a chance. When I read Gaskin's words, I get the sense of a sage trying to show us a way to creating new frameworks. Pointing us not to new answers but back down an ancient path to new questions. She is inviting us—women and men—to take a journey back to the source of our river, to see where else these same waters might take us.

I long for this book to be read not just by pregnant women but by all women, and indeed men. I believe we would do well to hold Gaskin's writings up among the great philosophical contributions of our time. I hope that this book will serve you as deeply as it has served me, in the creation of your families and beyond.

Ani DiFranco
September 2010

CHAPTER 1

The Importance of Birth and Birth Stories

Birth matters. It matters because it is the way we all begin our lives outside of our source, our mothers' bodies. It's the means through which we enter and feel our first impression of the wider world. For each mother, it is an event that shakes and shapes her to her innermost core. Women's perceptions about their bodies and their babies' capabilities will be deeply influenced by the care they receive around the time of birth.

No matter how much pressure our society may bring upon us to pretend otherwise, pregnancy, labor, and birth produce very powerful changes in women's bodies, psyches, and lives, no matter by which exit route—natural or surgical—babies are born. It follows then that the way that birth care is organized and carried out will have a powerful effect on any human society. A society that places a low value on its mothers and the process of birth will suffer an array of negative repercussions for doing so. Good beginnings make a positive difference in the world, so it is worth our while to provide the best possible care for mother and babies throughout this extraordinarily influential part of life.

Birth also matters because the journey through pregnancy and birth offers an irreplaceable way for women to explore their deepest selves—their minds, bodies, and nature. Such a journey of self-discovery can help them prepare for the hard and underappreciated job of motherhood in a world now full of historically unique and complex challenges. There is a sacred power in the innately feminine capacity of giving birth. It is one of the elemental, continuing processes of nature that women have the chance to experience, and it is the one act of human creation that is not shared by men. Why would we not want to explore this territory?

My use of the word "sacred" as applied to birth in this book is intentional and nonreligious. It implies that birth is an event important enough to warrant special consideration from those who are involved in the care of women during this time of life. It indicates that disrespect of the power of giving birth creates profound disharmony and ignorance in the world.

Giving birth can be the most empowering experience of a lifetime—an initiation into a new dimension of mind-body awareness—or it can be disempowering, by removing from new mothers any sense of inner strength or capacity and leaving them convinced that their bodies were created by a malevolent nature (or deity) to punish them in labor and birth. Birth may be followed by an empowering joy, a euphoria that they will never forget, or by a depression that can make the mother a stranger to herself and everyone who knows her. There is an enormous range of "birth effects," depending on each woman's experience, her lifestyle, the state of her health during her pregnancy, the choices she is able to make regarding the maternity care available to her, and the way she is treated when her time comes.

Traditional cultures throughout the world have always considered birth to be within the domain of women. Because only women give birth, indigenous cultures that were widely separated from each other all considered it obvious that women were the people most qualified to decide what sort of care was necessary during pregnancy, birth, and the newborn period. Even in those tribal cultures in which men had important roles to play around the time of pregnancy and birth, women—and in particular, those serving as midwives—had (and in some remote places still have) a great deal of influence in mapping out what these male roles ought to be.

What a contrast there is between these kinds of assumptions and those that are entertained by much of the public in the US. Here and in a growing number of countries, women have very little, if any, decision-making power about how they will be treated during pregnancy or birth. These are the countries in which midwifery either doesn't exist anymore or is so marginalized as to be without influence. This kind of extremely medicalized maternity care has become common in urban areas of Mexico, Brazil, China, Venezuela, and Thailand, for example, where rates of C-sections have risen to four or five times more than the rates considered safe by the World Health Organization (WHO). In 1985 and again in 2007, the WHO convened consensus conferences to review scientific evidence on technologies used in childbirth. These conferences made a series of recommendations, including that the rate of C-sections should never be more than 10 to 15 percent of all births.[1] Many private hospitals in the countries mentioned above have cesarean rates of 90 to 95 percent. The doctors who were my mentors during the 1970s would have been horrified to know that such high rates of surgery could be allowed to happen for no medical reason in any country, because they knew that unnecessary surgery puts lives at risk—the opposite of what medical care is supposed to do.

Just after I was given a tour of a birthing room at a high-volume Brazilian hospital in 2004, I had a chance to witness a scheduled C-section. The nervous husband of the mother-to-be and I peered through the window in the door of the operating room as we stood in the corridor outside. Trembling with fear, the mother lay on the T-shaped operating room table, her arms outstretched and tied to the table at her wrists. A nurse quickly shaved and swabbed her belly. There were no words of comfort given the mother through her ordeal. It seemed clear to me that while she was terrified of having the C-section, she must have been even more scared of experiencing labor or she wouldn't have agreed to the surgery. This hospital did have a birthing room, but I was shown the log of births that had occurred in it for the previous month, and only two women had made that choice. Several hundred others had opted for C-sections that were rarely medically indicated. I found myself wondering if this mother knew anyone who had given birth the way her grandmothers or great-grandmothers had. She must not have known that it could be within her capability to give birth vaginally without harm to herself or her baby, or that a joyful birth was a possibility.

Watching her, I remembered the lecture on birth that I had been invited to give to a roomful of psychology students in Brasília a couple of days earlier. Each one of the women students who were mothers had had C-sections. When I told the class that it was possible for women to give birth vaginally without anesthesia and to enjoy such experiences, most looked at me in disbelief. When I showed them a photo of an unmedicated woman giving birth with a look of ecstasy on her face, only the men in the class had the courage to look at it. Several seemed interested in knowing more. What took me aback was that each of the women closed her eyes and refused to take even a glimpse of the photo, even though I had assured them that the woman had required no stitches and lost no blood during the process of giving birth. Unlike some US women of the same age whom I had previously shown the photos, these young Brazilian students had become so deeply afraid of giving birth that any sense of curiosity about how this woman's body had accomplished it was overwhelmed by fear and a superstitious and unquestioning faith in technology. That's real fear.

While it is true that in several of the countries with high C-section rates many healthy women are actively choosing to have C-sections that aren't medically necessary, it can be argued that in the majority of such cases, their choices aren't truly choices because they are based upon superstitions about technology and surgery, coupled with erroneous assumptions and fears about their own bodies and the process of birth. The same goes for those women who submit to choices made by their husbands or other family members,

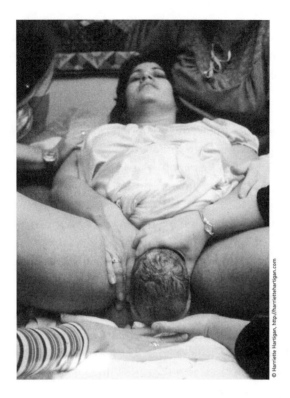

and those who have been persuaded by popular media and rather recent cultural fashions with no scientific basis that C-sections are safer than vaginal birth. In most cases, this is not true, and C-sections come with greater dangers for mother and child. It is time for people to be educated about this fact. Too much surgery is dangerous, and this is one of the reasons for the relatively high maternal death rates in the countries mentioned above. In contrast, countries that trust the natural process of birth and where midwives attend most of the births have better results. Finland, Iceland, Norway, Denmark, Sweden, the Netherlands, Belgium, Germany, the four countries of the United Kingdom (UK), and at least twenty-eight other countries all do better in this respect than we do in the US, although even these countries are being affected by the increasing use of birth technologies that tend to undermine the confidence of many women in their innate ability to give birth. When cesarean surgery becomes the norm for birth, maternal death rates inevitably rise.

We now find ourselves in a situation in the US and in many other parts of the world where women are increasingly being denied what is perhaps the most powerful and primal experience a woman can have: the right to give birth without the use of medical interventions unless these prove necessary. Women have been taught to believe that they must sacrifice themselves in important ways in order to have a baby—that the greater good for the baby means that the mother must submit herself to greater risk, even if that means a C-section for which there is no medical reason. For instance, many women are taught to think that it is automatically dangerous to a baby to be born vaginally if the cord is wrapped around the neck, when in fact almost all babies with the cord around the neck (per-haps one-fifth of all births) can safely be born vaginally. Others are taught that there is something so inherently dangerous about being forty-two weeks pregnant that justifies the induction of labor, even though that often leads to a C-section; in fact, an "estimated due date" is a guess that turns out to be wrong more often than most people realize.

My intention in this book is to call for greater involvement of women in the formulation of maternity care policy and in the edu-cation of young women and men about birth. Women who are fully informed about the capacities of women's bodies should lead the way, and all women who care about social justice and human rights should be involved. The way a culture treats women in birth is a good indicator of how well women and their contributions to society are valued and honored. Of course, fathers, husbands, brothers, and all other men who care about the women in their lives need to be involved as well. This should happen in every country, but it is par-ticularly important that the involvement of a partnership of mothers and midwives be increased in those countries in which there are either too few of the interventions that are sometimes needed during the process of birth or too many of these interventions, because both kinds of system errors cost women their lives.

I do want women who have already had C-sections to know that I am not judging them for having had surgical births. I understand that there are a lot of complicated reasons for having C-sections, and I make it a point to refrain from sitting in judgment on other women's choices. At the same time, much of the information that is dispensed about C-sections is incomplete or distorted, and this can lead to women making choices without all of the facts.

The latest figures indicate that all is not well with motherhood in the US—the maternal mortality rate has risen sharply in some states at the same time as maternity care costs per capita have escalated to levels two to three times as high as those in nations of comparable wealth. Some of our cities have maternal death rates that are worse than those in countries with far fewer resources; Costa Rica, Cuba, Bulgaria, Croatia, Hungary, Macedonia, and Slovenia are just a few examples of countries that are spending their resources designated for maternity care in a better way.

My intention in this book is not to persuade those women who want to avoid pregnancy to change their minds—far from it. But I do want to convince even women with no interest in motherhood that the right to a positive and safe birth is just as important as the right to choose whether or not to have a child. I do think that there is great value in taking a deeper look at motherhood and trying to discover what it might have to do with women's empowerment. We need to deepen our understanding of where we have been as women in the past and how the past has shaped and often distorted our knowledge of our bodies and ourselves, especially in the realm of pregnancy and birth.

The natural birth philosophy that had its origins in the 1950s and 1960s in the US and continues today in many countries around the world is based upon a fundamental respect for nature that recognizes that nature mostly gets it right in birth. According to this philosophy (I'm actually more inclined to say "observation"), pregnancy is not an illness in need of treatment, and nature's design of women is not considered flawed. The late Professor G. J. Kloosterman, an influential and eloquent Dutch obstetrician, perhaps said it best when he wrote: "By no means have we been able to improve spontaneous labor in healthy women. Spontaneous and normal labor is a process, marked by a series of events so perfectly attuned to one another that any interference only deflects them from their optimum course."[2] Such a philosophy, of course, does recognize that a pathological or dangerous complication can occasionally develop even in healthy women, and that the application of a powerful technology (surgery, for example) can be lifesaving in these instances. However, it excludes the introduction of powerful technologies either preventively or preemptively.

The guiding principles of the Coalition for Improvement of Maternity Services (CIMS) explain the natural birth philosophy quite well:

- Normalcy: treat birth as a natural, healthy process.
- Empowerment: provide the birthing woman and her family with supportive, sensitive, and respectful care.
- Autonomy: enable women to make decisions based on accurate information and provide access to the full range of options for care.
- First do no harm: avoid the routine use of tests, procedures, drugs, and restrictions.
- Responsibility: give evidence-based care used solely for the needs and in the interests of mothers and infants.[3]

Another set of principles related to natural birth was drawn up at the International Conference on Humanization of Childbirth held in Fortaleza, Brazil, in 2000. These principles fill out a vision of a better way for babies to be born:

- Humanized birth means putting the woman giving birth in the center and in control so that she, not the doctors or anyone else, makes all the decisions about what will happen.
- Humanized birth means understanding that the focus of maternity services is community-based (out-of-hospital) primary care, not hospital-based tertiary (specialist) care.
- Humanized birth means midwives, nurses, and doctors all working together in harmony as equals.
- Humanized birth means maternity services that are based on sound scientific evidence, including evidence-based use of technology and drugs.[4]

Women who share the natural birth philosophy want the opportunity to labor in a way that emphasizes human connection rather than monitoring by a machine. They know that surgeons and medical technology are necessary sometimes but not infallible, and that, given the realities of human greed, ambition, impatience, institutionalized ignorance, and gullibility, it makes sense to trust the processes of one's healthy body over the promises of miraculous cures and remedies—no matter how respected and authoritative the source may apparently be. As the late indefatigable researcher and writer Barbara Seaman put it, "Some women want to let their doctors do the worrying for them. But for those of us who don't, it has been extremely difficult to get honest health information."[5]

THE IMPORTANCE OF BIRTH STORIES

The influence that birth has on a society is powerful, but it's also subtle, because most of its initial effects are laid down in the private spheres of human activity in technological societies—in hospital maternity units, birth centers, and, more rarely, homes—out of the sight of most people. Because of its private nature, birth is much more mysterious to civilized people than it is to people who live in cultures in which birth occurs in homes and villages where encouraging stories are still shared about pregnancy and birth, and members of the village not only witness labor and birth but celebrate it collectively. In the same way, people in urban cultures no longer have the chance to observe the chains of cause and effect that emanate from each pregnancy and birth. The result of this is that most of us don't have direct ways of knowing how much variety there is in the ways women can give birth, without risking or endangering themselves or their babies.

As long as I have been writing and lecturing about birth, I have found it helpful, even necessary, to tell positive birth stories. This is one of the best ways for women to learn the kinds of things that may help or hinder labor and birth. Stories teach in memorable ways. In that sense, they are much more valuable than rote learning and memorization.

Stories have always been a medium of education amongst humans. When I encounter a story that reveals something about labor or birth that is new to me, I don't automatically dismiss it as untrue or irrelevant simply because I am unfamiliar with the phenomenon it reveals. In some cases, I have learned that the cultural blindness that highly industrialized societies have developed surrounding birth keeps us from observing behavior that used to be commonly known and is still commonly known in areas of the world where women retain control of birth.

A story that I heard from a friend before I had ever even witnessed a birth served as this kind of eye-opener for me. This was Jane's first pregnancy, and her baby was due any day. She was one of those women who trusted her body and felt strong and able to be on her feet doing things, no matter how pregnant she was. She and her baby's father were working in different parts of the city that day, and she didn't know until day's end when she rejoined him at home that he had had to leave work early because of violent abdominal cramps that had made him wonder for the next several hours if he had appendicitis. That concern was abandoned, however, when Jane's massage of his belly rather quickly quelled his pain. Shortly after both had eaten a meal, she began to experience cramps and thought she might have a stomach flu. Worried that this flu might start her labor, she decided to sit on the toilet, in hopes of finding some relief there. Within a few minutes, she cried out to him, "Come help me! Everything's coming out!" When he came running, their baby fell into his father's waiting hands. That was the first time I had ever talked to someone who gave birth without realizing that she had been in labor.

Hearing Jane's story reminded me of what I had read about couvade (from the French for "hatching or brooding"), the term used by anthropologists to describe customs from tribal societies all over the world that recognize that the psychological ties between parents-to-be during labor and birth are deeper than civilized people believe possible. In one typical account, an anthropologist described the phenomena he observed among tribal people of the Congo, noting that as the mother's labor begins, her husband apparently falls ill, complains of stomach pains, and loses his appetite. "Men know the instant of the birth of their children because at that instant their symptoms disappear," wrote the anthropologist. "A few men suggest that these symptoms may be due to worry about wife and child, but numerous cases are also cited in which a man is far away from home, falls ill suddenly, recovers just as quickly, and then learns of his wife's delivery at these very moments."[6] This account closely matched Jane and her husband's story and that of a birth I attended some years later—the fourth birth for a couple that I had helped before. In this latter case, unlike their three previous labors, during which the mother had experienced the sensations of labor, the father-to-be was the one who felt the pain of labor. This was not an act for either of them, and none of us could analyze why it happened for them in this way when it hadn't for their previous three births, but the father's pain left just as soon as their baby daughter was born. What was significant for me about both of these cases of couvade was that none of the parents involved had ever heard of the phenomenon before experiencing it.

While stories can't let women know what their own experience will be like, they can illustrate how wide the range of normal behavior is. Melissa, who lived next door to me while I was getting my bachelor's degree in literature, told me one that I found valuable. She was a tiny woman with a husband who towered over her. It's worth remembering, by the way, that in those days, unless you were a medical or nursing student, there weren't any books or photographs available to prospective parents of what labor and birth look like. When Melissa was nearly ready to give birth, her belly looked impossibly huge to me, and I worried for her. I wondered how the baby could possibly get out. I remember her stopping by my place before she left for her doctor's office for what she hoped would be her last prenatal visit. About three hours later, she returned home with her baby in her arms. "What happened?" I asked, amazed that she could have already given birth.

"Well," Melissa said, laughing delightedly with her accomplishment, "My doctor examined me because he thought that might tell him when I might start to have the baby, but the exam put me right into labor, and she was born in only twenty minutes. I couldn't even get my socks off!"

That story was an eye-opener for me, but I didn't doubt a word of it. It was pretty deeply ingrained in midwesterners like Melissa and I not to exaggerate. I was so excited to learn that a woman could give birth as easily as an animal that I forgot about how improbable it had looked to me a few hours earlier. Melissa's story and her eyes, shining with excitement and accomplishment, showed me what was possible for a woman who had never given birth before.

There had been almost nothing to read about birth in the libraries that I had access to as a teenager, but I did find Dr. Grantly Dick-Read's classic *Childbirth without Fear*, which I devoured at the age of sixteen. From it I learned something that rang true to me: much of the pain experienced by women in birth can be attributed to fear and to a lack of knowledge about the true physiology of birth. Fear leads to muscle tension, which can lead to more fear and increasing muscle tension unless the cycle is broken. Part of what made Dick-Read's book interesting was that he told personal stories about painless births he had witnessed—births that had completely surprised him because he had previously observed and therefore assumed that all births had to be extremely painful. Witnessing those painless labors prompted him to drastically rearrange his ideas about birth and to incorporate ways of educating women in how to lessen fear of birth and pain. He recommended deep, slow breathing during labor and other techniques for achieving a state of calmness and deep relaxation. He said that women who led sedentary lives would have more difficulty giving birth than peasant women who lived and worked outdoors. "The office worker tends to have more trouble than the fisher-girl, the farmhand or the riverboat woman," he observed.[7] He provided ways for urban women to overcome any difficulties caused by a largely sedentary lifestyle. Another recommendation he made—one that I subsequently found helpful both in my own labors and while assisting other women in labor once I had become a midwife—must have stuck in my mind from that first reading of his book. It had to do with the forehead muscles of a laboring woman, and it was this: women who could completely relax their facial muscles would be able to go through labor with maximum ease. I still find this advice to be useful and true. What I didn't know until much later was that most obstetricians in the US and the UK (Dick-Read's country of origin) during the sixties were far from comfortable with his ideas and methods. Their discomfort with his theories probably stemmed in part from the fact that his book was addressed to women, not to his fellow physicians, but it's also safe to say that most obstetricians are skeptical upon hearing that labor and birth can be experienced without pain, fear, or pain-numbing medications. It's not easy for surgeons—and it's important to realize that obstetricians are surgeons—to have a chance to witness such births. In fact, as I'll explain in more detail later, it's not possible for most US maternity nurses these days to witness a physiological labor that is allowed to proceed without intervention, either during their training or when they are employed in a maternity ward.

As a medical student, Dick-Read was also used to witnessing births that were extremely painful, so he was surprised the first time he had the opportunity as a medical student to observe a painless birth. As he describes in *Childbirth Without Fear*, it happened in a dingy tenement in the outskirts of London in 1911, and the only sour note during the entire labor came when the laboring woman turned down his offer of anesthetic gas. "It isn't supposed to hurt, is it, Doctor?" she asked him when he inquired afterwards why she had refused his offer. A few years later, his stint as a battlefield surgeon during World War I gave him the chance to see two more such labors, both of which took place outdoors near the surgical tents where amputations and other operations were carried out. Neither woman spoke English, but each made it clear that she chose to be near medical help just in case she had a complication, but that she didn't want anesthesia or to be told what to do. Each woman very calmly delivered her baby and placenta without any assistance and then picked up her baby and walked away after a few moments of rest.

Still another story taught me how Native Americans recognized the spiritual and emotional needs of women and their families around the time of birth. I got a glimpse of what the sanctity of birth meant in a practical sense in 1978, when some of the people from my community in rural Tennessee took part in the Longest Walk, during which Native Americans from all over the country walked from California to Washington DC. The Walk was a national demonstration organized to protest and lobby against several bills before Congress that a coalition of tribal leaders felt would further weaken treaties and land rights. When it reached Ohio, a young woman in early pregnancy began to miscarry and one of my midwife partners drove her to a local hospital. Once the miscarriage had happened and she was able to leave the hospital, she asked for but was refused her baby's body. According to her people's traditional practices, she needed to bury her baby with the proper ceremonies. However, she and my partner were unable to convince anyone at the hospital to release the body to them, because according to mainstream US culture, her baby hadn't yet reached the stage of viability, so was not entitled to burial. When the mother and my friend returned to the encampment and Ernie Peters, chief of the Walk, and the other elders were told what had happened, it took them only minutes to gather up a delegation of men to drive to the hospital to reclaim the body. This time, whatever was said quickly convinced hospital officials to release the tiny body, and the proper ceremonies and burial were performed before the walkers resumed their eastward journey. I wondered how many women belonging to the mainstream culture who suffered miscarriages would have appreciated some sort of cultural recognition of their loss—the kind of attention this Native American woman received after hers. I knew that I would have.

NOTES

1. World Health Organization, "Having a Baby in Europe," *Public Health in Europe* 26 (1985): 85.
2. G. J. Kloosterman, "Why Midwifery?" *The Practicing Midwife* 2, no. 2 (Spring 1985): 5-10. See the text at www.inamay.com/?page_id=249.
3. For further information on the Coalition for Improving Maternity Services and its mission, see www.motherfriendly.org.
4. M. Wagner, "Fish Can't See Water: The Need to Humanize Birth," *International Journal of Gynecology and Obstetrics* 75, supplement (2001): S25-37.
5. Barbara Seaman, "Dear Injurious Physician," *New York Times*, December 2, 1972.
6. Judith Goldsmith, *Childbirth Wisdom from the World's Oldest Societies* (Brookline, Massachusetts: East West Health Books, 1990).
7. Grantly Dick-Read, *Childbirth Without Fear: The Principles and Practice of Natural Childbirth* (London: Pinter & Martin Ltd., 2005), 192.

Second-Wave Feminism, Birth, and Motherhood

Nothing is so firmly believed as that we least know.
—Michel de Montaigne, *Essays on Divine Origin*

The sacred feminine is very closely related to women's ability to give birth. This has been true throughout human existence. Archaeological finds such as the Venus of Willendorf of Austria; the Venus of Lespugue of France; the *sheela-na-gigs* of the Irish and British Isles; the pregnant goddess figures of central Europe; and the birth figures of Latin America, among others, confirm that the creative power of the birth-giving woman was given honor and respect in cultures in diverse parts of the world.

It is interesting then that second-wave feminism, as expressed in the US during the sixties and seventies, was largely scornful of the status of women of indigenous cultures and assumed not only that all women in such cultures were victims of patriarchal systems but also that there was no expression of female power within them. The general view was that women who lived without access to modern technology had little or no real power. Some influential feminist voices that were otherwise quite insightful almost exclusively saw motherhood as a trap to women's advancement, one that should be avoided by whatever means possible. References to babies as "parasites" and phrases such as "baby pollution" were commonly heard, and anyone who advocated for more natural ways of giving birth than was the norm in the seventies was considered by many to be a traitor to her gender.

I learned this for myself on a memorable occasion. Asked to speak briefly about my work in midwifery to an auditorium of Yale students in the midseventies, I showed a couple of slides of mothers and their newly born babies from my community and was surprised at the immediate and vehement chorus of boos and hisses that came from the young women present. Instead of seeing midwifery as a means of female empowerment, these young feminists were repulsed by the very idea of birth. If anyone in that audience had the slightest curiosity regarding that subject, the auditorium was not a safe place to express a question. For this group of young women, who were, as far as I could tell, pretty representative of the philosophy that was prevalent on college campuses at the time, the only worthwhile choice was to avoid motherhood by any means necessary.

My idea of feminism included a wider spectrum of reproductive choices than these young women's ideas did—that was clear. I was in agreement with the idea of birth control, even though I wasn't impressed with most of the methods being championed at the time. I had already tried using an intrauterine device (IUD), but had it removed because I couldn't put up with the constant cramping and the overly heavy periods it caused. I was afraid of using the Pill, as I knew that it would alter various systems of my body in ways that hadn't been adequately studied. I've always resisted being a human guinea pig. Besides that, out of the first fifteen or so births I attended, about half were birth control failures of various kinds. I didn't want to put any poison inside myself to avoid getting pregnant when it might not even work, and I didn't want to participate in new methods that I knew were still experimental.

I supported the legalization of abortion, and I was sure that it was better that it be legal than for women to put their lives at risk with back-alley procedures. At the same time, I knew from talking to many of my friends who had had abortions that many women got them not because they really wanted them, but rather because they had been abandoned by the baby's father and by their own families.

These women didn't have a fair choice either, and their voices were not being heard. Because of that, for more than a decade my midwifery partners and I offered an alternative to abortion for women who didn't really want one by providing them with free room, board, and maternity care at our midwifery center. If they wanted to leave their baby with us for foster care, we arranged that, and if they later wanted to come back to reclaim the child, we also made that possible. Most of the three hundred or so women who took advantage of this service decided to keep their babies.

I had expected that young Yale women would be as excited as the women in my midwifery community and I were to learn that healthy women's bodies work much better than people in the US commonly believed, and that women could feel empowered in how they gave birth. What appalled the Yale women, I think, is that those women in my community were not seeking the kind of empowerment that was measured solely in masculine terms, apparently the only kind of which the Yale women had the least awareness. Like the Brazilian women I was to meet later, they were too frightened and disgusted by birth to be able to think clearly about it.

The idea that true feminists should not give birth seemed a bit daft to me. It reminded me of the philosophy of the Shakers, a communal group with branches in England and the US that was founded in the eighteenth century and believed that everyone should be celibate (the only way to avoid giving birth during the eighteenth and nineteenth centuries). Shakers were historically known for their gender equality and contributed much to US culture by way of their architecture, their fine furniture designs, their inventions, and their songs and dances. However, it is hard to keep a movement going when the only ways of adding members are adopting orphans and recruiting. By the time of my Yale visit, the only surviving members were a few old women. Of course, second-wave feminists of college age around 1970 weren't planning on celibacy—far from it.

The Native American women I knew, on the other hand, had very different views about women's empowerment and reproductive rights. Because sterilization without consent was a big issue for them during the seventies, reclaiming women's right to give birth as their foremothers had was an expression of both personal and cultural sovereignty. I talked to several women who had C-sections in hospitals on reservations and were sterilized without their consent at the same time, so escaping unnecessary C-sections was also a good way to escape an unwanted tubal ligation. Because they were furious that the right to give birth had been taken away from them, motherhood seemed like anything but a trap to them.

During the seventies and early eighties, our midwifery center at The Farm became a place where Native American and African-American women could get a taste of how a move back to midwifery could be empowering for them. The Farm is the name of the community that my husband, Stephen, founded in 1971 with the help of 270 people, most of whom had attended his Monday night classes in San Francisco during the previous four years. We traveled as a caravan across the country before settling in Tennessee and establishing a community on some forested land we bought. At any rate, the Native American and African-American women who spent some weeks or months with us were interested in serving the women of their communities, expanding their choices and thus freeing them from the discriminatory or often neglectful or insulting treatment so many were enduring in the hospitals that were available to them.

NATURAL BIRTH ON THE FARM

If the Yale students I spoke to had witnessed the powerful and euphoric births I observed at The Farm, I think they would have felt differently about the relationship between birth, motherhood, and empowerment. If any of them had already given birth in a US hospital, perhaps they would have had a better understanding of what we were about. Beginning in the early seventies, I was able to learn midwifery in a way that was self-directed and did not interfere with natural processes. Having experienced the US hospital birth treatment for the birth of my first child, a regime which called for a weight gain of no more than fifteen pounds (my obstetrician had me taking diuretics every day, something that I later understood to be quite risky) and a mandatory episiotomy and forceps delivery (the latter simply because I was a first-time mother), I decided that such treatment could not have been scientifically valid and began to educate myself about other possible options. I later learned that the rate of forceps use in the area where I gave birth the first time was an incredible 65 percent of all births.[1] (When Europeans hear of such rates, their jaws tend to drop in disbelief.) Some US obstetricians, when pressed to explain why the rate was so high, blamed it on deficiencies in US women's bodies. According to this explanation, European populations were ethnically and racially homogeneous, so European obstetricians didn't have such high rates of forceps use, while the US population was so heterogeneous that most US women produced babies with enormous heads that could not fit through their mothers' pelvises. I had traveled in Europe and hadn't noticed any difference in the size of people's heads and women's pelvises, so I found that explanation absurd and unscientific. At the same time, I knew that inserting forceps did not reduce the size of a baby's head or increase the size of a woman's vagina, except by seriously injuring one or the other—and sometimes both.

I won't relate the story of how I became a midwife here, since it is included in my first book, *Spiritual Midwifery*, except to say that I had the timely help of a kindly obstetrician and, later on, three family physicians. These doctors set a standard for me about what physicians ought to know and about the importance of the compassion that each demonstrated in the way he treated women in his care. I also had an extraordinary chance to work with and learn midwifery from a few hundred pregnant women who were living in The Farm's community with me, and I was free to recruit from this group the women whom I wanted as my midwifery partners. Over the years, many older obstetricians encouraged me in my quest to develop a more caring and respectful way of caring for women in birth. These gentle men, sweethearts every one, derived joy from assisting at births and, in most cases, had had their medical education in circumstances that allowed them to observe the full course of labor without intervention. Sometimes they spoke in sadness about how obstetrics was changing in ways that took the joy out of the occasion for everyone involved, and they lamented the loss of manual skills that are no longer being taught to physicians in training.

At any rate, counting from the first birth I ever witnessed—which occurred in a school bus camper in a parking lot at Northwestern University in Evanston, Illinois—186 babies were born before the first C-section was necessary. The second C-section was the 324th birth. No one died because of our relative inexperience during the early years of our practice, but had my two assistants and I not received an early seminar in appropriate emergency response to birth complications from Dr. Louis La Pere, my wise and good-hearted obstetrician friend, things could have gone differently. After Dr. La Pere's seminar, I knew how (and had the proper equipment) to resuscitate a baby who failed to breathe just after birth, how to deal with an umbilical cord tightly wrapped around a baby's neck, how to stop a maternal hemorrhage, and other vital skills. With the obstetrics handbook that he gave me, I began my studies of human birth and all the ways that humans have devised for dealing with this life transition.

I was able to learn midwifery in a way that permitted me to closely observe the birth process in hundreds of women without any imposed rules that would have interfered with the flow of labor. This was quite unusual for that time, and it allowed me to observe phenomena and cause-and-effect relationships that medical, nursing, and hospital-based midwifery students would rarely (if ever) observe. I could see, for instance, how quickly a terrified woman could become calm and unafraid if the right action was taken or the right words spoken. I could see how previously unbearable levels of pain could diminish in the same fashion. The women in my community were happy to have unmedicated births in their own homes, and I was under no orders to keep them from eating or drinking during labor, to keep them from taking a nap during labor before pushing their babies out, to keep them from moving around during labor, or to make sure that they had their babies within certain time limits. As long as the vital signs of both mother and baby remained within the normal range, the mother was unafraid, and there were no early signs of a complication, our practice was to allow labor to continue. Because I had got through most of my first labor without any medication quite well (despite being forced to stay in bed) by pretending that I was a mountain lion, it made sense to me to help women think of themselves as competent animals, instead of insisting upon a notion of human exceptionalism. It seemed crazy to me to take on the belief that the human female is the only mammal on earth that is a mistake of nature. Whatever you might have heard to the contrary, we women are just as well made for giving birth as any other mammal. The fact that we walk on two legs instead of four does not hamper this ability. If we need to, it's quite possible for us to take a hands-and-knees position, which is much like being a four-legged mammal. And special interventions in the birth process should be no more necessary among human females than they are among other female mammals, as long as we humans are well nourished, fit, aware of how our bodies and minds work, and healthy. I repeat: we humans are not inferior to hamsters, rhinoceri, squirrels, or aardvarks in our reproductive design. It's our minds that sometimes complicate matters for us.

At any rate, this free way of learning allowed my partners and me to approach birth with what Zen teacher Shunryu Suzuki calls "beginner's mind." Like my favorite high school teacher, Mr. Leonard Cole, who advised his biology students to keep an open mind, Suzuki knew that it is desirable to maintain a readiness of mind that is open to everything. "In the beginner's mind there are many possibilities; in the expert's mind there are few," he wrote.[2]

My prior education had prepared me to become an English teacher or perhaps a writer (I had a master's degree in literature by this time), but hearing the stories of a few women who had given birth at home by coaxing a labor and delivery nurse into serving as their midwife inspired me and put me on a radically different track. I was going to become a midwife, if only I could find a way. At that time, however, I was not aware of any training program that offered this kind of education, and I had never met a midwife or known of any in the US. As I mentioned earlier, my interest in midwifery was sparked by the birth of my first child—an obligatory and unnecessary forceps delivery that left me feeling both violated and puzzled. I had expected kindness and respect in the maternity ward, but instead felt as if I was being punished for having had sex (the only way one could get pregnant at that time), and wondered why they felt it necessary to tie my arms down when I hadn't been disagreeable or abusive. When my dentist had removed impacted wisdom teeth a few years earlier, he had trusted me not to fight him while he was at work. Why was the relationship between doctors and women so different in the maternity ward? Why did it feel so much like a medieval torture chamber, and why did I have to pay for this insulting, inadequate treatment?

As it happened, the first birth that I had the opportunity to witness—the one in the school bus camper—taught me something that completely surprised me, because the laboring mother looked so radiant and beautiful as her body did its work. What I was seeing was the power and beauty that women emanate when they are able to trust the wisdom of their bodies to labor and give birth in a way that is undisturbed. From anything I had previously read, I had expected at least some expression of anguish, but there was none (as long as I followed Lisa's plea that I maintain eye contact with her). I had expected sweat and blood as well, but these, too, were missing on this particular occasion. What stuck with me is that I should do everything possible to help a woman look good during labor. I was certain that every woman giving birth deserved to be treated with love and tenderness and that such treatment would go a long way toward preventing bad things from happening. I am still sure this is true.

After the publication of my first book and several invitations to speak to medical students and residents at teaching hospitals, I was to learn that few obstetricians had opportunities to witness unmedicated labors that were not interrupted by routine interventions. This lack of experience usually left them with a distorted idea of what labor could be like without intervention. Instead of seeing women looking radiant and gorgeous as they labored, they saw terrified women with high levels of adrenaline who were in extreme pain. High levels of catecholamines such as adrenaline cause pain, and this development in turn causes more fear and thus even higher levels of pain. For these medical students and residents, every birth seemed to be an ordeal. I, on the other hand, was observing women with high levels of the ecstatic hormones—oxytocin and beta-endorphins, the latter of which is a powerful opiate produced by the body—in their system. Women who have had very painful experiences during labor and birth often don't think that they could possibly have experienced less pain if they had done something differently or if they had been treated differently, even when this is true. Unless they have a chance to witness another way of giving birth, they usually remain stuck in the idea that what they experienced was somehow inevitable.

At any rate, I was able to assemble a team of midwives, backed by Dr. John O. Williams Jr., a family physician who had a soft spot for midwives. Our C-section rate for our first four hundred births was 0.5

percent during a time when the national C-section rate was 5 percent of all births. (In 2008, the US C-section rate was 32.3 percent, nearly 5 percent higher than it had been only five years earlier.) Our rate of forceps use was 0.05 percent, which compared with rates nationally that varied between 40 and 67 percent. As a relatively highly educated group (during the seventies, we counted our university degrees and realized that we had more among us than did the members of the Tennessee legislature) who owned a big piece of land but had little money, The Farm was something of an anomaly in our rural area of Tennessee, where most women took it for granted that they would be unconscious or unaware during labor and that their babies' fathers would not be permitted to be present for labor and birth. However, our combination of talents, the hard-working lifestyle that we adopted, and our determination to win the acceptance of our Tennessee neighbors proved a winning combination.

Dr. Williams always acknowledged that providing maternity care for an Old Order Amish community near The Farm for many years not only added to his knowledge of obstetrics but also exposed some

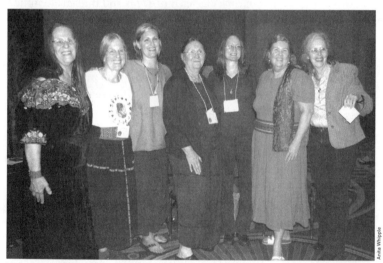

My partners and me: Sharon Wells, Pamela Hunt, Stacie Hunt, Carol Nelson, Deborah Flowers, Joanne Santana, and me.

of the myths surrounding birth as taught in the US. Doctors were routinely taught that women who had had more than five babies were at great risk for bleeding to death after birth, and that home birth put both mothers and babies at risk of infection. This conservative group used no birth control, so the average couple had about thirteen babies, most of whom were born at home. In spite of the many pregnancies each woman typically had, hemorrhages after birth were rare, and even though there was sometimes a fly in the house around the time of birth, the Amish mothers and babies rarely contracted infections, while the hospital nursery had to be closed several times during that time because of infections that swept through it. Dr. Williams told us that he thought that people tended to develop immunities to the organisms in their own environments, and that this explained why the Amish women remained healthy while giving birth at home.

BIRTH CULTURE AS DEVELOPED AT THE FARM

Fear plays a large role in childbirth in the US, and it is fed by ignorance. Knowledge is empowering because it is an essential step toward stepping away from fear. Women who think that their minds and bodies are separate from each other have little idea how much their thoughts and feelings affect the course of labor. It is usually difficult for midwifery, medical, or nursing students to learn such cause-and-effect relationships, given current hospital routines that create stress in laboring women, impose time and movement restrictions, and do not allow the students uninterrupted time with a single laboring woman who is being treated appropriately. In fact, I have met many nurses who had not a single chance to be in the same room with a laboring woman at any time during their training, but were then hired as obstetric nurses. This creates a situation that is far from ideal, since the nurse in this case is usually fearful and uncertain as to how to help the laboring woman.

I had a rather unique chance to witness the important relationship between fear and labor early in my career, when two healthy first-time mothers who had spent many hours with their cervices 75 percent open were only able to progress further when meaningful words that addressed their hidden anxieties were spoken. For the first of these mothers, it came to light after many hours of labor at The Farm that the mother, who had been adopted as a newborn, was afraid that her biological mother had died in childbirth. Immediately after this fear was revealed and quelled, her cervix (which had previously felt as if it was held in place by an embedded wire) opened completely, and she was able to push her baby out. I had no idea before this birth that mind and body could be so directly connected, but it was obvious that this was no mere coincidence. Grantly Dick-Read had not been exaggerating when he wrote that fear was the enemy of good labor.

The second woman had anxiety of a different kind—a fact that I learned after being with her constantly during nearly two days of strong labor. Her cervix had been seven centimeters open for more than a day, with no sign of opening more. I had never known of anyone who had had such a long labor, but her baby's vital signs and her own continued to be good—one guideline to which Dr. La Pere had stressed that I must adhere. That was reassuring, but clearly, something had to change. Finally, in frustration, I asked if anything was bothering her. "Actually, yes," she said. She explained that when she and her husband had married, they had written their own vows. She had wanted them to include a vow of lifetime commitment to each other, but he found that too morbid. Certain that this was the key to her problem but not knowing what might be done to remedy it, I asked Stephen what he thought. He suggested that if the couple were willing, he knew the traditional vows and could conduct an impromptu ceremony. They did agree, and once the couple had finished repeating their vows—interrupted by a couple of contractions—Stephen left, and approximately an hour later, the baby was born. After those two births, there could never be any doubt in my mind about the unity of mind and body, and this became the cornerstone of my practice.

During the months and years that followed, several women told me that expressions of love or praise from their husbands caused an immediate and noticeable dilation of their cervices. Another surprised me as I was checking her dilation by saying, "I just want to open up and have this baby now!" As she spoke those words, I felt her cervix open a significant amount. When I told her what I was feeling, her joy at hearing this enabled her to open even more. In this way, birth by birth, I was able to observe how women's emotions correlate with their bodies' ability to open during the process of labor.

SPHINCTER LAW

I was also able to learn that even after the cervix has opened a great deal, sudden fear, a painful vaginal examination, or even the wrong person entering the room can cause the cervix to close in many women. Usually, such a change will cause the intensity of the labor to lessen, but it's also possible for labor to come to a complete stop. This phenomenon of a complete reversal of labor was well understood by most medical textbook authors during times when home birth was the norm, but when birth moved into hospitals, and women were on "foreign" territory, maternity care became increasingly fragmented, and many doctors never had the chance to learn that their own presence could bring labor to a complete halt or even reverse cervical dilation.

One of the first stories I was ever told about a home birth taught me something that I have carried with me ever since. Ava's labor took place in a commune in which members were given no privacy, to the point that someone had even bothered to remove the bathroom door. She told me that she was sure that her labor would have been much shorter than the forty-eight hours that it actually took if she hadn't had to endure the presence of so many curious people. Hearing that story taught me the powerful effect that the presence of observers can have on a woman in labor. During my second year as a midwife, I encountered a case in which a woman's cervix opened to eight centimeters and then went back to four centimeters—a phenomenon that I had never read about in any medical or nursing textbook. The mother had been laughing and joking during most of her labor but had become rather serious as her dilation increased. After a few moments of consideration, I asked if she might reactivate her sense of humor and see if that change in mood might enable her cervix to open again. That strategy worked beautifully: her cervix reopened, and her baby was soon born.

I invented the term "sphincter law" to describe this phenomenon, because I thought it could help people who have never given birth to have a better understanding of how women's bodies function during labor. We all have sphincters and therefore have some understanding of how they are related to emotional states. Sphincters, of course, are the ring-shaped muscles that surround the opening to various organs, such as the stomach, the bladder, and the anus. The cervix, although not strictly speaking a sphincter, behaves like one. Basically, sphincters are shy, and they open better in privacy. They don't obey orders, because they are part of the autonomic (or involuntary) nervous system. Once they begin to open, they can suddenly slam shut when their owner is embarrassed or frightened. Many people have had the experience of being midway through a bowel movement in a public toilet when suddenly the expulsion process reverses itself upon hearing a fire alarm. This is part of the natural fight-or-flight response to perceived danger. Catecholamines (adrenaline) rise in the bloodstream when an organism is frightened or angered. Female animals in labor in the wild, such as gazelles and wildebeest, can be on the point of giving birth and yet suddenly reverse the process if surprised by a predator. Nowadays, it's possible to find films or videos on the

Internet of mammalian mothers in the wild whose babies are on the point of emerging when they are involuntarily sucked back inside in case of sudden danger. The same evolutionary behaviors take over in us humans when we go into labor, without our necessarily understanding the evolutionary wisdom of our own behavior. I know many women who have experienced this type of reversal during labor.

Because physiology is far more constant than is human culture, these phenomena take place every day, but few doctors, novice midwives, or nurses recognize what is happening. Medical textbooks no longer reflect this still valid knowledge, so when dilation is stalled or reversed, the woman is usually told that she has "uterine dysfunction," "inadequate contractions," or a mysterious condition called "failure to progress." In each of these cases, she is usually told that she must either have her labor augmented with intravenous oxytocin or have a C-section. Midwives in busy hospitals tell me that they often notice that when a shift change occurs when a woman is in strong labor, her dilation often lessens when the midwife she has become used to suddenly leaves and a complete stranger comes to her side. A by-product of this brand of ignorance that became entrenched in the US in the early twentieth century is that most medical personnel are no longer taught that many laboring women have a need for privacy and kindness that is similar to that of other mammals. Similarly, medical personnel are not taught that a woman who holds her mouth and jaw in a relaxed way as she pushes will have a better chance of getting out her baby without tearing as her baby emerges—provided that she is not being pressured to push too hard and too fast. Technology-induced ignorance is now spreading even to veterinary medicine, as several veterinarians have told me about people bringing their pets to "the hospital" when they go into labor. When they are told that the best thing to be done is to leave the animal alone for a little while, they protest and insist that the veterinarian "do something." Leaving the animal alone *is* "doing something."

The time limits that have been imposed on laboring women since the nineties have surely contributed to the rise in the C-section rate. The obstetrics handbook that was given to me by Dr. Louis La Pere in 1970 was one that most US doctors in training at the time would have owned. Author Ralph Benson, in the section "The Course of Normal Labor," wrote: "The first stage of labor may be less than 1 hour or *more than 24 hours*" (my emphasis).[3] At that time, when US C-section rates were about 5 percent of all births, the lack of regimented time limits on labor was one of the factors that made such low C-section rates possible. In the fifties, Dr. Emmanuel Friedman published a paper about a labor progress chart that he thought could establish "norms" for labor. According to his "Friedman Curve," every woman's cervix should open at a predetermined number of centimeters per hour, depending upon whether it was her first baby or not.[4] It is doubtful that Dr. Friedman foresaw that his paper would be used in the ways it was in the nineties, when being in labor became a race against time in many hospitals. The "Friedman Curve" was used to justify a great increase in artificially stimulated labors and a corresponding decrease in the number of hours allowed for laboring women to dilate. Currently, it is unusual for women to be allowed to labor for more than ten to twelve hours before the pressure is applied to go for a C-section. (According to this formulation, I would have needed five operations instead of the five vaginal births that I've had.) While I have seen plenty of labors which could be described by a Friedman-like curve, I have seen just as many whose graphs had long plateaus at the same dilation, followed by sudden increases to a higher dilation—labors that ended with the births of healthy babies.

We women are not machines. When labor proceeds in a way that is undisturbed, it often can't be described by a progress curve that would look satisfactory to an engineer. Even so, that doesn't mean that we are ill-designed. It just means that we have emotions and sphincters, not mechanical parts. One other little tip: laughing helps to open sphincters and to keep them open—more about that below.[5]

There is plenty of evidence that the presence of different hormones secreted by women's bodies during labor explains the phenomena that I described above. Adrenaline is the hormone that is active when a labor reverses itself or stops. Most people have some familiarity with the effects of adrenaline—it makes us stronger and faster, and it is the "fight or flight" hormone that is activated when we perceive danger. When adrenaline (catecholamine) levels are high in a laboring woman's body, her pelvic muscles will be tense, and she will experience much more pain than she would if someone were able to assuage her fears.

Most people know that oxytocin is a drug that is often given in synthetic form to women in hospitals to make labor stronger, or is given after birth to prevent or stop excessive bleeding. However, they are less likely to know that women's own bodies are capable of secreting oxytocin and that this endogenous oxytocin not only causes uterine contractions (and thus keeps labor moving along and prevents excessive bleeding after birth), but that it is associated with feelings of love, trust, gratitude, and curiosity. While synthetic oxytocin can be effective in stopping hemorrhage by causing the uterus to contract, it does not induce feelings of love, trust, gratitude, and curiosity in the way that the mother's own oxytocin does. In addition, synthetic oxytocin, when used for strengthening labor, causes more painful contractions that often lack the painless rest periods of unmedicated labor. When adrenaline levels are high, oxytocin levels are low, and vice versa. (These changes, by the way, can take place almost instantaneously.) The women who reported feeling their cervices open when words of love were spoken were responding to elevated levels of oxytocin in their bloodstream.

Dr. Kerstin Uvnäs Moberg and her team in Sweden carried out some of the most useful research of the late twentieth century in the area of maternal-infant behavior.[6] Their work effectively demonstrated that people's oxytocin levels rise significantly when they share a pleasant, delicious, and unhurried meal together, and when they are in the process of falling in love. But the highest levels of oxytocin of all occur in mothers and their babies during the first hour just following birth. This is the time of bonding, when mother and baby are programmed by nature to adore each other and share moments that neither will ever forget. Such moments should only be interrupted for medical procedures when a true emergency occurs; interruptions should not be routine. Interestingly, when such important moments are allowed to unfold without interruption, the risk of postpartum problems in mothers and babies is reduced. Babies breathe better and their heart rhythms are more regular when they have skin-to-skin contact with their mothers' chest. Mothers are less likely to hemorrhage in these circumstances as well.

Beta-endorphins are a third kind of hormone relevant to labor and birth. Beta-endorphins are nature's opiates, and they have powerful pain-numbing effects. When we expend a lot of physical effort, beta-endorphin levels rise correspondingly. They also rise when we are warm enough and, most importantly, when we are feeling secure. Being in love and feeling sexually aroused are also associated with high levels of endorphins.

I am well aware of how skeptical most people will be about the strength of beta-endorphins. Sports physicians, however, are well aware of the threat of reinjury when an athlete is playing well—the pain of a reinjury might not be felt because of the beta-endorphin rise caused by strenuous and successful play. People who have had to free themselves from traps in ways that involve the need for self-injury often report that they could bear the pain—another example of the potential strength of endogenous beta-endorphins. It is important to remember that fear and negative emotions inhibit a rise in beta-endorphins. This is one reason why whining does not alleviate labor pain, whereas moaning may. There is an important distinction between these two kinds of vocalization. Moaning is a sound that may indicate pain, but may also indicate pleasure, and is consistent with relaxation; whining indicates complaint and self-pity, is high-pitched, and doesn't happen during pleasurable experiences.

Beta-endorphins, combined with oxytocin, explain why some women—as strange as this may seem to anyone who hasn't seen or experienced it—experience orgasm during labor or birth. Orgasm, of course, is an experience that we almost exclusively associate with making love—so much so that some women become offended and upset even thinking about the possibility of having such an experience while giving birth. I think this kind of reaction has much to do with the fact that the medical model of birth has successfully wiped from most people's minds the obvious fact that women give birth with their sexual organ. Further confusion results because women in our culture are not taught that their vaginal tissues have the ability to swell in a way that is every bit as impressive (and surprising, viewed for the first time!) as the change in the flaccid penis when it becomes erect.

Every man knows that erections happen because of blood that is trapped in the penis. The penis enlarges far more than it could if it were forcibly and hurriedly stretched to its maximum. The trouble is that women don't have such an obvious way of knowing that vaginas do fancy tricks too and that blood can suffuse the vaginal tissues in a similar way in order to easily allow the passage of a full-term baby without tearing. High levels of both endogenous oxytocin and beta-endorphins are necessary for such swelling. Obviously, such hormonal levels are not possible when women are in great pain, feeling threatened, or being subjected to constant interruptions—just as men don't get erections when they're terrified or being threatened with sharp instruments.

Too many women have been exposed to the myth that when a baby passes through the vagina, that organ will be permanently stretched and ruined. It is true that vaginas can be badly injured when babies are pulled through with vacuum extractors or forceps, just as they can be injured by rape. However, when vaginas are treated well and are not subjected to routine episiotomy or forced pushing, they swell impressively, since these tissues have the ability to hold a large amount of blood when the mother's labor has produced the ecstatic hormones of oxytocin and beta-endorphins. Under these circumstances, vaginas function marvelously in birth, and when they become small again, they are no more ruined than is a penis when it softens and shrinks following an erection.

Very intelligent women can easily become so frightened by lack of information or by myths they have been handed early in life that they come up with some fanciful ideas about what is possible in nature. I learned this years ago from Mrs. Anna Mary Sykes, a midwife of my mother's generation who grew up in Arkansas. We had just finished watching several birth videos, and she turned to me and said, her eyes twinkling with amusement, "I never saw anything like that when I was growing up. When I was in labor with my first baby, I didn't even know where my baby was going to come out!"

"Is that right?" I said, half-amazed by her story but knowing that she wasn't exaggerating. She was clearly not a woman who would do that.

"They didn't tell us anything, even when we were getting married," she answered. "When I was still pregnant, I looked all over myself. I was trying to find out where that baby was going to come out.

"I had a mirror and was looking all over my body. When I opened my mouth, I thought that must be it. When I saw that little thing in the back [her uvula], I thought that was the baby's big toe. I thought I was going to have to throw up the baby. It wasn't till the midwife came and washed between my legs that I knew that was where the baby was going to come out!"

I had to think about that for a while, because Mrs. Sykes was the first woman of her generation to share with me the naïve fears she had developed from growing up in a culture that allowed her no knowledge about what happens in birth. That's fear of the body—

one's own body—in its rawest form, followed by a great leap of the imagination. If that was the baby's big toe, where was the rest of his body? Where were his knees? How could she swallow her food or get that lumpy body and head past her neck when it was time to "throw up" the baby? Denial, coupled with fear, makes for irrational thinking.

A couple of Amish grandmothers, each of whom had given birth thirteen or fourteen times, later confirmed that such irrational fears also occurred in some of their daughters. One told me, with amused eyes and a knowing smile, "It takes them a while sometimes to figure out that it's going to come out the same place where it was put in!"

THE INNER PRIMATE

One of my specialties during the early days of cultural development at The Farm was teaching "civilized," "educated" women how to behave like indigenous people—actually, like any other mammal. I often found it easier to take the shortcut of explaining to women that we all have an inner primate, and that this is the part of ourselves that we need to access when we are in labor. "Let your monkey do it" became the phrase I used to say to those intelligent, often competitive women who, by force of habit, used to try to "think" their babies out. I continue to find it helpful to introduce pregnant women who have the usual cultural fears about giving birth (how can something so big as a baby come out of my body without damaging me?) to their "inner ape" or "wild woman." It also seems to help them if they understand that optimum labor requires them to enter into a trance state—not a logical, thinking state.

With every successful birth, my midwifery partners and I gained a new ally in our teaching effort, because each woman now had an empowering birth story that she was eager to share with others. Free from legal, institutional, or professional constraints, we were able to create our own birth culture, and my partners and I were able to explore the question of what birth could be like if we combined the best knowledge from the ancient world with the best use of technology from the modern world. For us to stay out of the hospital as much as possible, we needed to teach women to be wild when they gave birth. It's actually quite gratifying to observe a woman with an MD, a JD, or a PhD hunker down and find her natural woman and realize she knows how to give birth as well as any orangutan on the planet. It's awesome.

But what about pain?

Everybody knows that it can hurt a lot to give birth to a baby without pain medication. It's not so well-known that some women do not experience birth as painful. Does this mean that every woman will experience a painless or almost painless labor? No. However, the fact that it is possible should make it clear that there is no automatic curse on women in labor. Probably the one and only generalization about birth pain that can be safely made is that women who have had painful births have trouble imagining a pleasant labor. Of course, the same might be said of a woman whose only sexual experience has been rape. She might believe it impossible for any woman to have a pleasant sexual experience. A patient, loving partner, and, possibly, skillful therapy may help a woman traumatized in this way to learn to let her guard down enough to find pleasure in a sexual act that previously only provoked extreme pain.

The very thought of pain scares a lot of women, in part because we associate pain with physical injury. One of the biggest myths about birth pain is that it is continuous for most women. It isn't continuous (unless labor has been augmented with synthetic oxytocin or some other uterine stimulant, or the dangerous complication of placental abruption is taking place). Usually, it lasts for less than a minute, and then stops for an interval of several minutes before the cycle starts again, with that interval usually becoming shorter as the woman moves further into labor. Because the rests between contractions are painless, the woman then knows that her body hasn't been damaged by what has happened so far. Additionally, there is a great deal of variation in the pain thresholds different women can handle. A study comparing a group of Dutch women's expectations of labor pain with those of a group of US women found striking differences. Both groups of women had hospital births and were asked the following questions within two days after they gave birth: What were their expectations of pain? Did they take pain medication? How would they prefer pain to be managed in a future labor? Both the Dutch group and the US group were informed of the potential negative effects of pain-relieving medications for labor. The US women *expected* labor to be more painful than the Dutch women did, and they expected to be given medication for pain. Nearly two-thirds of the Dutch group received no pain medication, in contrast with only one-sixth of the US women. In both groups, the proportions of women expecting pain to those who actually received medication were nearly identical.[7]

Perception of pain also varies greatly according to where women give birth. When I began hearing home birth stories for the first time in the late sixties, one common thread I noticed in the stories of women who had also had previous hospital births was that they remarked that labor hadn't been as painful at home as it was in the hospital. (Several reported there had been no pain during their home birth at all.) This phenomenon can be explained in more than one way: first, higher levels of ecstatic hormones can probably be reached when women are in the place where they feel most secure and comfortable (their homes), and second, women who labor at home are more apt to be in the position they want to assume, rather than the one they are asked to take.

Whatever the place of birth, the biggest enemy is fear, because fear itself can cause and accentuate pain. Women in labor are often very surprised to find out how much pain can be alleviated just by taking slower, deeper breaths. Those who are able to move around freely in labor instead of passively obeying when told to lie in bed find that moving can relieve a lot of pain. These actions help the laboring woman move into a trance state. Indeed, birth pain, as unlikely as this may sound to the uninformed reader, can be alleviated in many ways: by the presence of a calm, knowledgeable person (like a doula, or a certified labor companion), by immersion in warm water, by dancing, and by laughing. Laughing? Yes! Even a little smile immediately boosts beta-endorphin levels in the bloodstream, which numbs pain. Laughing helps even more, and it helps with the dilation of the cervix as well. (If you are skeptical about this, try this strategy if you are ever painfully constipated and are scared about splitting when it's time to poop.) All of these actions increase the secretions of oxytocin and beta-endorphins, which both facilitate birth. These actions also move the blood supply away from the forebrain and toward the bottom areas, where swelling needs to take place. And when it works better, it feels better.

What US women often don't learn about birth pain from books they read or births they see on television is that choosing a C-section simply to avoid pain means that they will experience it after their baby's birth rather than before. They often think, erroneously, that pain medications will remove all sensations of pain during the days following surgery. Millions of US women who have read a best-selling book about pregnancy and birth have encountered this statement: "Even though it is technically considered major surgery, a cesarean carries relatively minor risks—closer to those of a tonsillectomy than of a gallbladder operation, for instance—that can generally be treated easily."[8] That may be reassuring to many pregnant women, but it is far from the truth. Every abdominal surgery, including a C-section, is highly invasive, so the comparison with a tonsillectomy is completely unwarranted, and a C-section, unlike gall bladder surgery, can never be performed via laparoscopy (a minimally invasive technique). Everyone has pain after abdominal surgery, especially when sneezing, coughing, laughing, moving around, or attempting to stand up straight. Additionally, being mobile during the days following surgery is a necessary way for all postsurgical patients to reduce the possibility of forming blood clots in their legs, a potentially fatal complication. This risk, by the way, is elevated in women after C-sections, because of the high levels of clotting factors that are present in women around the time of birth—nature's way of reducing the risk of hemorrhage.

A TRUE WOMEN-CENTERED ETHIC

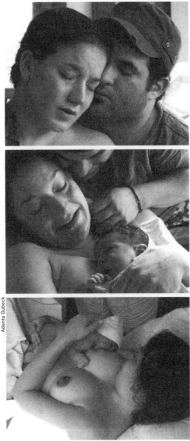

Adanta Qubeck, Luis Fernandez, and baby Ixaya.

The time is ripe for the development of a women-centered ethic in the US that includes the complex issues that surround birth and motherhood. A women's movement that is too narrowly focused to take seriously the needs of women becoming and being mothers is itself in a stage of prolonged adolescence and must mature. It is time for feminists to realize that pitting the needs of nonmothers against those of mothers is a way of weakening—not strengthening—women. Women should not lose their human rights when they become mothers. The status of motherhood is progressively lowered when women themselves have little understanding of the needs of women who give birth and of the abilities of their own bodies. It is also important for women to be aware of the historic role of midwives and how their changing roles have played out in parts of the world where the profession of midwifery was not eliminated, as it was in the US during the early decades of the twentieth century. When giving birth to a new life is discounted as a possible source of female empowerment and ability, we place immense burdens on virtually every mother in our society, while at the same time expecting each one of them to live up to the ideal of being the Perfect Mother. We can and must do better than that.

NOTES

1 J. P. Greenhill, *Obstetrics*, 13th ed. (Philadelphia & London: W. B. Saunders Company, 1965).

2. Shunryu Suzuki, Zen Mind, *Beginner's Mind* (New York: Weatherhill, 1973).

3. Ralph C. Benson, *Handbook of Obstetrics & Gynecology*, 3rd ed. (Los Altos, California: Lange Medical Publications, 1968).

4. Emmanuel Friedman, "Dystocia and 'Failure to Progress' in Labor," in *Cesarean Section: Guidelines for Appropriate Utilization*, eds Bruce L. Flamm and Edward J. Quilligan (New York: Springer-Verlag, 1995), 23-41.

5. See *Ina May's Guide to Childbirth* for a fuller discussion of sphincter law.

6. Kerstin Uvnäs Moberg, *The Oxytocin Factor: Tapping the Hormone of Calm, Love, and Healing* (Cambridge, MA: Da Capo Press, 2003).

7. I. P. M. Senden, M. D. van de Wetering, T. K. A. B. Eskes, P. B. Bierkens, D. W. Laube, and R. M. Pitkin, "Labor Pain: A Comparison of Parturients in a Dutch and an American Teaching Hospital," *Obstetrics and Gynecology* 71, no. 4 (April 1988): 541-544.

8. H. Murkoff, S. Eisenber, and S. Hathaway, *What to Expect When You're Expecting*, 3rd ed. (New York: Workman Publishing, 2002).

Charlotte at The Farm

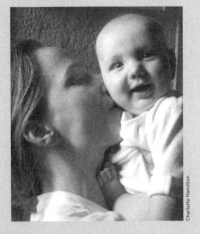

Charlotte Hamilton

We met Pamela in January on our visit to The Farm from our home in Brooklyn. I knew I had found the gentle, wise woman I had been craving to deliver our first baby. She included my husband Sam and specified how important the role of the father was going to be during the birth. My relationship to my baby "Ses" (he was sesame-sized when I took the pregnancy test) had been very sweet and unworried, and I wanted to give birth in the same way. To give myself the best chance for this type of birth, I chose to travel to this vegetarian community in the woods and surround myself with mothers, grandmothers, and midwives, many of whom had either given birth and/or been born at The Farm.

I arrived at Pamela's birthing cabin three weeks before the due date, and Sam arrived a week later. The cabin was cozy, and it was easy to feel at home. I loved waddling to The Farm's shop, talking with the sweet people I came to know over the next six weeks, cooking simple little meals and sitting at the table listening to the radio, being in silence most of the day. The birth cabin was next to Pamela's house, and when she went out she would always leave me with the phone number where she would be, telling me to call her if I started having contractions, or my water broke, or if I needed anything. One day she dropped me off a bowl of delicious salad on her way out, made with wonderful things mostly grown in her garden.

I went on four-mile morning walks and everyone I saw made me feel very much at home. I was spacey and meditative and had no need to "do" anything. People would smile knowingly at me and my belly, knowing I was doing my best to "walk the baby down." I spent time lying down, listening to sounds out of the window as I lay on the daybed. I didn't even want to read, just to move slowly in the heat and stretch my body a bit and then sit or lie down again. At night the cabin was enveloped by a loud chorus of chirping insects. I would leave the lights off to sit on the bed in the dark and look at the fireflies lighting up the forest, wondering when the baby would come, and if maybe these night sounds would be the very first thing he would hear.

I was big bellied and slow moving in the heat, and in the afternoon I would go the long route to the swimming hole to cool down and enjoy the sun and the dragonflies. When Sam arrived he brought more energy and together we explored further, picking blueberries at dawn or dusk, taking day trips to local towns. Together we kept quietly wondering when the baby was going to come and what it would be like . . .

At noon on the 22nd of July my water broke, and we began getting excited. I had to squat on a big pot and collect some fluid as it leaked out, and then pour it into a glass to have a good look to be sure that I wasn't leaking pee or something. Sam went out to let Pamela know. I sat cross-legged with my back against the wall and closed my eyes and told the baby I was ready for him and would do my best and that I loved him and wouldn't hurt him. Sam made potato salad and I moved about mostly in the bedroom on the bouncing ball and on my hands and knees, enjoying the thickness of the carpet. The contractions were pretty mild and fifteen to twenty minutes apart. I tried to eat a lot of food because I didn't want to get depleted later on. By 5:00 PM the contractions were seriously strong and five to ten minutes apart—I couldn't do anything but long, slow, and steady mouth exhalations. The intensity would be level, then increase and I would feel slammed until I "got" it, and knew to be ready for the next one. Pamela told me I needed to be more vertical to get him to come down so I stopped leaning forward. She told me to lean on Sam and get strength from him, and soon after I couldn't manage a contraction without him. From about 7:00 PM I had them every two to four minutes until the birth the next day at 9:15 AM, and it was crucial to have his strong, solid body to put my head on or his eyes to look into or his mouth to watch doing a long exhalation so I could keep going and not freak out.

I threw up a few times in the early evening and was sorry to see that food go down the toilet. It was as if both ends of me were erupting or convulsing or something. I kept using the bouncing ball, walking around and going in and out of the shower, where I'd lean my forehead into the wall and talk to myself in the dark: "I'm fine," "I'm doing it," "I love you, Ses," "This is happening," "I can do this," with the shower running on my lower back. I talked to myself that way the whole time, mostly just in my head but sometimes aloud. I also said "Help" and "Oh my God" a lot, and told Sam we are adopting the next one!

At 9:00 PM Pamela checked my cervix and it was five centimeters dilated. I was lying on the bed for that and I was a bit surprised that it wasn't time to push already! I was very glad to get off my back; even for those few contractions it had been excruciating. A few hours later I was in the birthing tub. As I leaned my head on my arms with my body stretched into the water I saw outside the fire of a citronella torch, red flames glowing in the night sky. I felt as if I was being both acknowledged and protected. My body was a very intense place to be by this point. I had nowhere else to go, and the rate and continuity of the contractions really amazed me. I didn't figure out how to rest effectively in the tub, but would hang onto Sam's shoulders or arm and make him help me breathe. "Calm down," I told myself between contractions, "You're okay, calm down." I sipped water and coconut water through a straw. I'd get up to go and pee every now and then. It would take several separate movements between contractions to get to the toilet and back.

At 2:00 AM Pamela suggested I try lying on my side on the bed. She said the contractions would get more intense but there would be bigger gaps between them and I would be able to rest between them better. I did lie down beside Sam for a few of them but was pretty blown away by how hard they were. I got on the ball for a bit and held onto Sam as he lay on the bed. We both dozed between contractions, and if he was still sleeping when one came I would squeeze him and gasp for help. They just carried on getting stronger and stronger, and at some point I was back in the tub. It was hard to communicate about the temperature of the water because it was almost impossible to talk even though my mind was very lucid and thoughts were crystal clear. Pamela checked my cervix and it was nine and a half centimeters dilated. I was so involved with the tectonic shifts happening within me. It felt like force fields and pulsations that could move mountains, all within my pelvis. Stacie, another farm midwife, came just after that at 4:30 AM while I was still in the tub. Pamela lay down for a rest in the sunroom and Stacie sat on the daybed—both of them were within ten feet if we needed them, but were giving us plenty of space too. I felt totally sustained by the baby I loved so much and the support of my husband, who stayed with me through every contraction. I had started lying on my side in the tub with my hand on my hip, trying to push it away from me. I thought I was making more space for the baby somehow, but Stacie said to try and push into the pain instead of trying to escape from it. I told Stacie I had to get out and go and poop; she said "No you don't, that's the baby's head coming down," but I went anyway.

The whole time they trusted me to know what I needed. Something about the dark of night and the warmth of the tub was too much like sleepiness, so I started moving between the shower and the toilet.

Around dawn Pamela went home to brush her teeth and came back with fruit toast and eggs. I was so glad they were eating, and I ate some peach and some toast. Pamela opened the cabin's doors and put a fan outside the front door to draw the fresh air in. It felt like kindness that the day had come and light and air, and as I lay in the tub I asked Pamela, "What do the next few hours look like?" She said the baby would be out before midday. "Oh sooner than that, definitely," said Stacie, "You are getting very close." I had started to wonder where the heck the finish line was, and I was very glad to hear that this epic did have an end in sight.

They brought a birthing stool into the cabin because I was erupting into grunts and felt best on the toilet. I remember as I sat on the stool Pamela looked me in the eye with her clean, gentle, strong face and said, "Okay Charlotte, it's not going to be a picnic from here on in," and I took strength from that. I was between the shower, the toilet, the birthing stool, and the birthing tub for the next few hours. I said to myself "Oh, OK, this is opening." Stacie and Pamela helped to stretch my cervix to get the anterior lip unstuck. Animal noises would explode out of me and I'd think "Christ, you have got to be joking," and then I'd hear Pamela and Stacie, serious and enthusiastic, telling me, "Good Charlotte, real good." When I was on the birthing stool Pamela said to pull up on the stool (the one bar forms a U-shape that you both sit on and hold onto) with my arms and push, using that to push my whole body down. She showed me where exactly to push into with my hands. I was strengthened, knowing I was working on an exit strategy for Ses. I remember thinking "Pull using my arms? Brilliant, I have strong arms. I can do this." Not long after my arms were shaking like wings, a visible sign of how maxed out my body was, whereas the internal journey for me cranking open and pushing Ses out was felt but not seen. I made a lot of noise, but Pamela told me to hold my breath instead and push all of that energy down instead of out my mouth. Later on Stacie again suggested I push into the pain to get it to move, that I would go through it to the other side. I tried and found it to be true—that in hunkering down into it, there was a rush of lightness.

At 8:30 AM I got the birthing stool in the shower and sat in there with Sam beside me, Pamela kneeling on the floor in front of me, and Stacie seated on the toilet. Pushing with all my might and pulling up on that bar, I could see my arms shaking like mad. My mind said, "Come on baby," "I love you," and "You can do it." My head would hang down and I would stare at the shower drain and its beautiful, orderly black holes. I could hear the voices of everyone, and I knew what they were doing and took in what they were saying, but all I could look at was the drain. I couldn't believe how huge this thing felt coming out of me. I joked with Pamela that no wonder people say it's the happiest day of their life: "Sure there's a baby, but even better, labor is over!" She told me that rest is on the other side of this. I could hardly believe it was ever going to stop. After so many hours with no break for more than a few minutes, this journey felt so real. He wasn't out yet, but we all knew how close it was, and there was happiness as well as exhaustion. Pamela said later that she had to make a judgment call at that time; she knew I was going to tear a little if I didn't take a few more hours, but she decided I was too tired to last that much longer. When I felt that baby's head thickly making its way down, I also knew I really needed it to be over. I got more energy to do some of those crazy, huge pushes. The crowning was at 9:05 AM, and they coached me through the pushes until finally, with the most wonderful feeling in the world, like every single hot, solid organ in my body was coming out together, my deepest, darkest, hugest bodily parts . . . a yelling baby boy was born at 9:15 AM. Pamela immediately had him in my lap covered in a towel, and I heard water pouring out of me into the shower and couldn't believe how happy I was to let my body go and just feel that little person. I thought he was huge, and understood why it was so hard to get him out, and did not understand how he had ever fit inside me. Pamela said, "Let's get you lying down." That was just the best thing I had ever heard. Lying on the bed, I could see Sam holding the little one in the rocking chair. My whole body felt like jelly and I relished the joy of having done it, having it be complete. I couldn't get over the happiness of how hard and massive and huge that whole thing had been and that I had done it.

The placenta wasn't making its own way out, and I felt too tired to know how to really push anymore. Pamela suggested I go and sit on the toilet where sometimes it just "plops out." I was there for only a minute; Stacey suggested putting the baby on my nipple, so Sam did, and then, plop, there the placenta went. I took a shower and got all the blood off of me, then lay on the bed so Pamela could do a couple of painless, careful stitches. Stacey sat next to her at the foot of the bed, Sam came in with the baby, and we all joked together and were pleased and proud of each other.

Knowing we were all exhausted, Pamela brought an amazing lady named Marilyn into the cabin to be with the baby so we could sleep. The cabin was calm, clean, silent. The work was done and we just absolutely loved being able to have a nap. Gilbert was lying in the sun being stroked from nose to tailbone with one finger, as Marilyn sang him folk songs and lay beside him. Sam and I slept deeply for hours.

We stayed in "our" cabin for two more weeks, which to me was as important as being there for the birth. Pamela checked in with us every day. She would smile and simply ask, "Do you have any questions?" She took our well-being and our capacity to thrive for granted, and in so doing set us on a steady, strong, and trouble-free path to parenthood. We were always reassured and admired and positively encouraged. I had fallen madly in love with Pamela by now, of course! Those first weeks were so precious, sleeping all the time, resting when awake, being fed huge, delicious meals by Sam, being vulnerable and loved, raw and clean, awestruck and present. I am glad for all of our sakes that we decided to have the birth in our cabin in the woods with Pamela at The Farm. If I am ever lucky enough to be pregnant again, I'm heading for Tennessee.

—Charlotte Hamilton

CHAPTER 3

Sexuality and Birth

Mainstream US culture teaches people that pregnancy and birth are illnesses for which hospital treatment is necessary. This cultural conditioning shapes people's thinking about labor and birth in ways that few question. Nothing could be less sexual than feeling ill or being in a hospital. Coming from this perspective, it would seem unusual—possibly even weird—for anyone to think of there being the slightest link between sexuality and birth.

But there is one way that our mainstream culture acknowledges birth as part of women's sexual lives, and that has to do with how birth is depicted on television. At the present time, the only kind of birth footage that can be aired without digital "draping" at the moment of birth is the C-section. When birth first began to be shown on US television during the nineties, decisions were made in broadcasters' boardrooms that it would be acceptable for people to see an incision made in a woman's abdomen and uterus and a baby's head be pushed through that incision, but not to clearly see a baby emerge from a woman's capable body, from her vagina. This kind of censorship in the service of "modesty" has the effect of teaching the public that the C-section is safer and more socially acceptable for mother and baby than a vaginal birth. *It also reinforces the notion that the woman's body is something that she should be ashamed of.*

In ancient cultures, the sight of the vulva of the goddess was a sacred image; our culture has made it taboo. However, the physical reality remains. Women give birth with their sexual organ; that is how we are created. Here is the contradiction inherent in the view that birth and sexuality have nothing to do with each other; in fact, how can sexual feelings not enter into birth, given its physical realities?

I, like most people raised in the US, never made the obvious connection between sexual feelings and birth until I witnessed a laboring woman whose husband was sitting at her side pull him closer and passionately kiss him during a long contraction. Her relaxation during this intense part of labor was instant and impressive: I could feel it in my own body. A feeling of calm confidence pervaded the birth room. This was an "aha" moment for me, because I realized just then that my own social conditioning had prevented me from imagining how much a little making out might help not only to augment labor but to numb pain at the same time. The ecstatic and beautiful birth that resulted from this woman's pulling her husband to her for a kiss—a real consciousness-changing kiss, mind you, not just a peck—enlarged my growing collection of practical techniques to pass along to other couples when it was culturally appropriate to do so. However, more than a year passed before I gave anyone that prescription.

The occasion was the labor of Aniana, a friend who had had two previous hospital births that had been terrifying for her. She mentioned the painful stitches she had had to recover from after each birth. This third labor, her first that was unmedicated, was proceeding rapidly, and the feeling of fear in the room was increasing with every second. Having already exhausted every helpful bit of advice that I had in my bag of tricks, I could see that both she and her husband were panicking, and I needed some way to calm her as quickly as possible. Just then the kissing couple came to mind, so just before the next contraction began, I suggested that Aniana try kissing her husband through it. It couldn't hurt, I thought, and might help. She nodded and turned toward him, first pressing her lips tightly together. He mimicked what she did, and they mashed their tightly held lips together for the duration of that contraction. Perhaps they were feeling self-conscious, but I knew something had to change for the kiss to be effective. Silent until the contraction was over, I suggested that when the next one came along, Aniana should try again but that she should open her mouth enough this time to surround her husband's. (I had already noticed at many births that women who held their mouths open as their babies were born rarely if ever suffered lacerations—as above, so below). The difference was instantly palpable: the panicked feeling disappeared and was replaced with ecstasy. The baby was quickly born over an intact perineum, which was particularly gratifying, as he was his mother's biggest. Years later, Aniana wrote me that the prescribed kiss and the birth experience that it made possible actually helped her marriage. She mentioned that their previous sex life could have been better, and that the kiss during labor proved to them both that deep, satisfactory connection was real for both of them.

People who are in denial about the possibility of sexual feelings during labor forget what happens in the body during a good kiss. Blood rushes from the thinking part of the brain, the neocortex, to the vaginal tissues, and this is precisely what causes the swelling that enlarges the vaginal opening enough to make painless penetration possible. Oxytocin and beta-endorphin levels soar. When a woman gives birth, she has—if anything—an even greater need for such swelling to take place. When her labor can proceed in a way that allows the release of high levels of oxytocin and beta-endorphins, the optimal swelling of her vaginal tissues can then take place. As mentioned earlier, the release of these hormones explains why some women—as strange as this may seem to anyone who hasn't seen or experienced it—experience orgasm during labor or birth.

A woman who wrote about her birth experiences in an online comment section about orgasmic birth explained how during the same labor, a woman might experience both pain and orgasm:

> My first birth, while excruciatingly painful thanks to back labor from a malpositioned baby, still left me

feeling on the verge of orgasm as he was born. My second unmedicated birth was completely pain free until my water broke at 9c (he was born 30 min later). Yes, ladies, pain free! In either case, I have never felt so aware of my body and its power as I did then. All my friends talk about how awful their births were. They were unprepared and not well-informed, so they followed the hospital protocol of staying in bed, strapped to monitors, at the mercy of doctors and their interventions. Every single birth plan was one word: epidural. But it doesn't have to be that way!! Birth is not something to be afraid of. It's not something to endure. Yes, it hurts—but pain is not going to kill you. We are too quick in our society to offer panaceas for anything uncomfortable.

Why aren't people in our society allowed to see what this looks like? I think it would be good for women to learn that nature provides the goods for such work. Seeing is believing, after all. Women who have been taught to be afraid of their bodies are easy to manipulate into making reproductive choices that they may later regret. The best way to combat fear is to provide accurate information that takes account of the wide range of phenomena that can occur. If every pregnant woman could see how the relaxed mouth and jaw, combined with pushing from the most effective position for any given woman (whatever that might be) and the slow emergence of the baby can make for birth without the smallest scratch in most women, the amount of fear that so many women feel would be noticeably reduced. If it's all right for little children in the US to listen to television commercials around dinnertime every night with lines such as, "If you experience an erection that lasts more than four hours, see your doctor," I think that those same little children's minds wouldn't be too badly bruised by seeing a baby emerge from a woman's body—at least on videotape.

Smooching, by the way, is one strategy for helping labor along that can be used wherever birth happens. Several British couples who gave birth in hospitals told me that they found it an extremely effective way of getting less sympathetic midwives to leave the room, while drawing the kindest one to their side.

THE *SHEELA-NA-GIGS*

For millennia, traditional cultures all over the world have created images of birth-giving women. Taboos like those that exist in our modern culture obviously did not exist in many indigenous cultures. It's interesting to consider the *sheela-na-gig* images that were carved in stone on castle walls or over Christian church doorways in the British Isles. It seems likely that most towns and villages there displayed such images in public places about eight to nine hundred years ago. As the centuries passed, however, an understanding of the original purpose of the images was lost, and many archaeologists have been at a loss to explain why they were ever made. The greatest concentrations of those that have survived were found at or near early Christian monasteries. Records show that it was the custom for brides to look up at the *sheela-na-gig* set high up on the wall of a church as they entered it to be married.

Whatever their form and size, I am sure that the *sheela-na-gigs* were made for the same purpose that I use them for: to quell the fears that young women can have when they are unable to imagine how their baby can be born. A visual image seems to help some women give birth more easily—a fact that midwives long ago surely realized, just as I did. I remember showing a first-time mother with my hands how much her body would open during birth, and she surprised me by opening more before her baby was actually pushing against her than I had ever seen before in a first-time mother. (Everyone who has attended births for women who have already

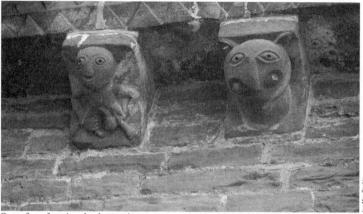

One of my favorite *sheela-na-gigs*.

given birth a few times know that their vaginas often swell and open before the baby presses them open). When I later asked her how she had accomplished this feat that I had never before known was possible, she told me that with every push, she had held the image in her mind of how huge she was going to get.

Surely, I wasn't the first midwife to ever notice this phenomenon in women. Some of the stone carvers who produced these images must have been instructed by the local midwives as to the postures, facial expressions, and hand positions of the *sheela-na-gigs* that they were to create.

I spoke with a woman in Edinburgh who told me that her Irish grandmother said that she had put a drawing of a *sheela-na-gig* up on her wall every time she was near to giving birth. A British midwifery colleague and friend, Sara Wickham, on hearing my interpretation of the social reason for the existence of the *sheela-na-gigs*, gave me a small ceramic replica of the first one I had ever seen pictured, on a stone church in Kilpeck, Herefordshire, near the border between Wales and England. I took it to a few births with me, and couldn't fail to notice the power this small image had to reassure women that their bodies could be capable of such a transformation during labor and birth.

In May 2010, I finally had a chance to visit the Kilpeck *sheela-na-gig*. For years, I had tried to picture how the figure was situated on the church and how the sight of it might have affected people about nine hundred years ago. I have always found this particular *sheela-na-gig* rather cute—even sweet—and seeing her in the setting where she was placed so many years ago reinforced this impression. This *sheela-na-gig* is one of about eighty figures on the corbel of the church, including some bearded masks, stylized animal faces reminiscent of the totem masks of Northwestern indigenous Americans, and some animal faces were so cute that this quality had to have been intentional. This was a church that children must have approached with delight, as they looked up to see these images, including the *sheela-na-gig* with her open legs, her wide-open eyes, and her curious half-smile.

Will modern-day Irish and British people come to view these images again without the puritanical overlay that caused explorers during the Victorian period to describe them as "ugly," "repellent," "immoral," "horrifying," or "threatening"? One of the *sheela-na-gigs* was described as "a shockingly crude, naked female with splayed legs and fingers holding open a gaping vulva. Two odd breasts, one with two nipples, a triangular Celtic head and a pipe-stem neck . . . whose attitude and expression conspire to impress the grossest idea of immorality and licentiousness."[1] This particular *sheela-na-gig*, and many others, show the hand or hands in the perfect position to touch the clitoris, a gesture that many women will instinctively make as their babies are being born. Just as men know that touching the penis in the right way will make the blood rush to it, some women seem to realize this just when they need to know it, while giving birth. For the rest, the *sheela-na-gigs* on the churches must have given them the right idea.

SEXUALITY AS AN IDEAL WAY TO INDUCE LABOR

It was impossible to be a midwife in my community and not to know that women often reported that their labor began right after love-making. These same women often reported that this was their favorite way to go into labor, as it made for "mellow," rather easy labors, as they described them. Years later I ran across an article in a medical journal that mentioned the large amounts of prostaglandins that can be found in human semen—there was a chemical basis for the phenomenon that we had observed (and experienced ourselves) so often.

When I talk to audiences of expectant parents about this, the fathers-to-be are usually happy to learn that they can be of service in this way. I like to remind people that this type of prostaglandin is effective at ripening the cervix near the end of pregnancy, that it carries with it no danger of overstimulation of the uterus (as do synthetic prostaglandins, which are often used for cervical ripening or induction), and that it is very inexpensive.

HOW SEXUALITY WAS ERASED FROM BIRTH
IN THE WESTERN MIND

When male physicians first began to attend births in growing numbers on both sides of the Atlantic, most births were still taking place at home. In order for male physicians to be accepted at that time, they had to convince the men of means who would be paying their fees that their instruments would provide an extra measure of safety for their wives and that it was not true that "decency was kicked down stairs, and modesty put out of countenance" by their presence at births, as one doctor-author wrote in the eighteenth century.[2] Male physicians had to convince husbands that there was nothing sexual about vaginal examinations, so safety became the dominant theme of the sales pitch. One Boston doctor argued in 1820 against a proposal to bring midwives back, commenting, "There can be no doubt that the attendance of a female must be more grateful to these feelings [of honor, virtue, and dignity], and that they must be somewhat wounded at first by the presence of a physician."[3] Dr. Hugh L. Hodge of Pennsylvania, who was clear in his mind that only men should attend births, came up with a formula that worked wonders for his cause. It would be necessary, he reasoned, to teach people that giving birth was *always* dangerous. This would sweep aside all the criticisms concerning women's modesty:

> If these facts can be substantiated; if this information can be promulgated; if females can be induced to believe that their sufferings will be diminished, or shortened, and their lives and those of their offspring, be safer in the hands of the profession; there will be no further difficulty in establishing the universal practice of obstetrics. All the prejudices of the most ignorant or nervous female, all the innate and acquired feeling of delicacy so characteristic of the sex, will afford no obstacle to the employment of male practitioners.[4]

As it happened, it wasn't even necessary for the doctors who followed Hodge's plan to substantiate the facts. It was easy enough to scare incoming medical students, other doctors, nurses, and middle-class Americans with overwrought prose, always pretending that this was science. Joseph B. DeLee, for instance, wrote several textbooks for doctors and nurses during the early twentieth century, in which he described the horrors that were inevitable if forceps weren't used to pull out every woman's firstborn:

> Labor has been called, and still is believed by many to be, a normal function. It always strikes physicians as well as laymen as bizarre, to call labor an abnormal

function, a disease, and yet it is a decidedly pathologic process. Everything, of course, depends on what we define as normal. If a woman falls on a pitchfork, and drives the handle through her perineum, we call that pathologic-abnormal, but if a large baby is driven through the pelvic floor, we say that is natural, and therefore normal. If a baby were to have its head caught in a door very lightly, but enough to cause cerebral hemorrhage, we would say that it is decidedly pathologic, but when a baby's head is crushed against a tight pelvic floor, and a hemorrhage in the brain kills it, we call this normal, at least we say that the function is natural, not pathogenic.[5]

And:

Can a function so perilous that, in spite of the best care, it kills thousands of women every year, that leaves a quarter of the women more or less invalided, and a majority with permanent anatomic changes of structure, that is always attended by severe pain and tearing of tissues, and that kills 3 to 5 per cent of children—can such a function be called normal? Much depends on what should be defined as "normal" for the human. Among insects it is the rule for the female to die soon after reproduction. The salmon invariably dies after spawning.[6]

DeLee's specialty, whenever he wanted to make a controversial point, was use of the questionable analogy. It's illogical to compare the reproductive behavior of women with that of insects or fish, since neither of the latter gives birth to live young. But medical textbook and journal editors, if they existed in those days, apparently had no problem with an author advocating a drastic new intervention and basing his entire argument on a glaring logical fallacy. It should be said that every DeLee prophylactic forceps delivery involved making a cut of several inches through the skin and muscles of the perineum, the area between the vagina and anus. Having been abused by such treatment myself, I was flabbergasted the first time I read DeLee's argument for the routine forceps delivery and realized that it had been his written words surviving years after his death that led to this cruel and crazy intervention during my first delivery. DeLee's influence was still so strong in the midsixties that more than two-thirds of all births were forceps deliveries in the area of the country where I was living. I felt raped after that doctor was done with me, and I proved three times (by giving birth to three bigger babies) that his forceps hadn't been necessary. Now that's a bad spell if there ever was one! There certainly wasn't anything scientific about the DeLee prescription for forceps deliveries.

The realization that sexuality and birth are related makes defunct the cultural myth that women's feelings (or, according to Dr. Hodge, the "prejudices of the most ignorant or nervous female, all the innate and acquired feeling of delicacy so characteristic of the sex"[7]) have nothing to do with their well-being or that of their baby during labor and birth. It is precisely because birth is sexual that women need to be treated with tenderness and compassion as they go through this extraordinary life passage—not fear and a routine forceps delivery. I know that my midwifery partners' and my recognition of the sexuality of birth has been a major factor in achieving good outcomes for the births that we have attended since 1970.

NOTES

1. John O'Donovan, "Ordnance Survey Letters" (Co. Tipperary, typed copy), *Royal Irish Academy Proceedings* 11 (1840). Quoted in James O'Connor, *Sheela na gig* (Tipperary, Ireland: Fethard Historical Society, 1991), 6.
2. Philip Thicknesse, *Man-Midwifery Analysed: And the Tendency of That Practice Detected and Exposed* (London: R. Davis, 1764).

3. Walter Channing, *Remarks on the Employment of Females as Practitioners in Midwifery* (Boston: Cummings and Hilliard, 1820). Quoted in Jane Donegan, *Women & Men Midwives: Medicine, Morality and Misogyny in Early America* (Westport, Connecticut: Greenwood Press, 1978).

4. Hugh L. Hodge, "Introductory Lecture to the Course on Obstetrics and the Diseases of Women and Children, Delivered in the University of Pennsylvania, November 7, 1838" (Philadelphia: J. G. Auner, 1838). As quoted in Jane Donegan, *Women & Men Midwives: Medicine, Morality and Misogyny in Early America* (Westport, Connecticut: Greenwood Press, 1978).

5. Joseph B. DeLee, "The Prophylactic Forceps Operation," *American Journal of Obstetrics and Gynecology* 1 (1920): 34-44.

6. Jospeh B. DeLee, *The Principles and Practice of Obstetrics*, 5th ed. (Philadelphia: W. B. Saunders Company, 1928).

7. Hugh L. Hodge, "Introductory Lecture to the Course on Obstetrics and the Diseases of Women and Children, Delivered in the University of Pennsylvania, November 7, 1838" (Philadelphia: J. G. Auner, 1838). As quoted in Jane Donegan, *Women & Men Midwives: Medicine, Morality and Misogyny in Early America* (Westport, Connecticut: Greenwood Press, 1978).

CHAPTER 4

A Brief Look at the History of Midwives and Medical Men

It is necessary to go beyond commonly held myths and to know at least some broad outlines of the history of women's health care in the US if we are to have any ability to shape coherent, workable policies for the future. It's impossible to make great plans as to where you are going if you don't know where you've been. Most people in the US have little understanding of why birth knowledge and policy evolved the way it did in the US and Europe, and they know just as little about the role that our national lack of midwives played in this evolution or why and how the midwifery profession was essentially eliminated for several decades in the mid-twentieth century.

One of the most intriguing mysteries surrounding the physiology of human birth is the vast gulf between what we might call the most basic knowledge base of midwives and that of most obstetricians. I'm referring to very different knowledge bases gained and taught in different ways that distinguish the midwifery model of care (a wellness model) from the medical model of care (an illness model). For four centuries physicians have been educated to view women's bodies as machines that often malfunction, to view pregnancy as an illness, and to view birth as a life-threatening problem that often requires surgery or instruments to save mother and baby.

In a broad and fundamental sense (and crude as this sounds), midwifery knowledge is based upon continuous observation of living women during pregnancy, labor, and birth, while medical knowledge from its early beginnings was based upon meticulous study of the bodies of dead women and babies. Once the church's prohibitions against the dissection of human remains were lifted in the late fifteenth century, the practice of dissection became the foundation stone for the later development of Western scientific medicine.[1] Dissection allowed medical men to name the organs of the body, an activity that lent them much prestige and allowed many to consider their knowledge superior to that held by midwives, who ordinarily didn't perform dissection. Anatomists could study the ways that babies had to rotate during labor in order to move through the pelvis. Such studies were useful for understanding the reasons for certain kinds of obstructed labor resulting from a baby being in a difficult position, but they were not helpful at all in understanding how to help babies in difficult positions be born, or in understanding how a change in the mother's position could facilitate the downward passage of the baby—things that midwives had learned empirically.

Men's solutions to birth complications have tended to focus on the creation and use of tools to solve problems, while midwives traditionally used a wide variety of ways to bring about the changes they wanted to see. Whereas a medical man might think of inserting forceps to pull out a baby that wasn't optimally positioned or moving through the outlet of the pelvis rapidly enough (sometimes they would even use them before the cervix was completely open, which can cause great risk to mother and baby), midwives would be more likely to ask the woman to move her body in such a way as to change the baby's position to a better one, or to help her find a position other than the obligatory supine position that doctors have nearly always favored. Belly dancing, for example, is just one way that certain cultures have devised over time to lower rates of fetal malpositioning during the last three months of pregnancy, or even to change a baby's position during strong labor.

John Maubray, an nineteenth-century English textbook author, exhibited the typical disconnect that took place between medical men and midwives when he complained about the methods those "obstinate creatures" (the midwives) were apt to use in a difficult labor.

> [The midwives] cram their patients with cordials, keeping them intoxicated during the time they are in labour, driving poor women up and down stairs, notwithstanding their shrieks, and shaking them so violently as often to bring on convulsive fits on pretence of hastening their labours, laughing at their cries, and breaking wretched jests upon the contortions of the women, whose torments would make a feeling man shudder at the sight.[2]

Maubray obviously had no idea how both the woman's movements up and down the stairs (lifting her legs for each step) and the shaking of her body (which can relieve pain but which obviously looked violent and painful to him) can correct the alignment of a baby who may be aimed at an angle that makes further descent difficult or impossible. He also had no appreciation of how much bawdy humor can assist a woman, not only in lifting her mood, but also in helping her cervix to open fully because of the beneficial hormones that humor can elicit in a laboring woman.

A German American doctor of the late nineteenth century, George Engelmann, was more observant than most medical men. In his book *Labor Among Primitive Peoples*, he made some interesting observations about the differences between indigenous and civilized women's abilities to labor well. After a colleague commented upon how indigenous women almost never assume the lying down posture that civilized women had come to believe the only one possible (or ladylike) for them, he commented on those who will squat and those who will not:

We may, in a general way, consider all postures as squatting which resemble that assumed in defecation. Though apparently inconvenient, and repugnant to the refined woman, this position is certainly the most natural one for expulsion from the abdominal or pelvic viscera, and will certainly, in many cases, facilitate labor. Thus a friend relates his experience: A colored woman, a house servant, carefully reared, who had undergone several very difficult labors, in her fourth or fifth pregnancy, feeling a little uncomfortable and desiring to be ready, took a pail and went to a pump for water. She carried it for twenty or thirty steps, and arriving at the gate, felt violent contraction. She set the pail down, squatted, and was delivered of her child.

He was so impressed, the following couplet occurred to him:

So easily she yields her bosom's load
You'd almost think she found it in the road.[3]

The problem for Western medicine has been that few medical men were aware that a living woman's pelvis is very different from that of a dead woman. The four bones of the pelvis of a living woman are able to flex and move in relation to each other, while the pelvis of a woman who has died is fixed in size and shape. This means that the internal shape and diameters of the pelvis change significantly according to the position taken by the woman and by the degree of flexion of her legs at the hip. When she lies on her back, for instance, the distance between her pubic bone and her tailbone and sacrum is significantly reduced. This can make it difficult or impossible, in some cases, for a baby to pass through unless the mother changes her position. When she adopts a hands and knees position, the diameter between the front and the back of her pelvis increases, a fact that was missed by most Western male medical authorities but which is better understood within midwifery tradition and knowledge worldwide.[4] I often suggest to pregnant women that they go to the Internet to watch the movements of large mammals as they give birth. One of my favorite sites is "The Dramatic Struggle for Life" at YouTube.com; it shows an elephant giving birth in an animal park in Bali. It is perfect for showing the perineal swelling that takes place when the female mammal is undisturbed and unafraid, the way she shifts her weight from foot to foot as she labors, and the dramatic opening of her mouth as she hunkers down when her baby begins to emerge from her body. Another strength of this video is that it shows the mother figure out how to stimulate her baby to breathe, a feat she accomplishes without having taken a course in neonatal resuscitation or having any human interference other than her captivity. (It's only fair to warn you, though, that the puritans at YouTube.com might ask you to verify that you are over eighteen if you want to see this video).

FLAWED PHILOSOPHY TAKES HOLD IN WESTERN THOUGHT

It didn't help Western knowledge of sex and birth that most medieval authors who mentioned women's bodies adopted the standard view that while men and women shared a common physiology, men's reproductive organs were perfect and women's left much to be desired. According to this perspective, a vagina was an inverted penis that had never fully developed. Themes of disgust and revulsion of the female body occupied many early writers' attention, including that of Saint Augustine, who offered these sentiments in the late twelfth century: "Concupiscence is a vice . . . human flesh born through it is a sinful flesh," and "We are born between feces and urine." Plato himself had opened the door to this kind of weird thinking when he asserted that the superior gods had created the head, while the inferior gods created the lower body. According to this view, the function of the human neck was to guard the head against the lower regions.[5] Plato was an upper class Athenian, served by slaves, so he never had to look out for food, or for his own safety. Plato's pupil, Aristotle, had this to say: "The female is, as it were, a deformed male; and menstrual discharge is semen, though in an impure condition; i.e., it lacks one constituent, and one only, the principle of Soul."[6]

De Secretis Mulierum (On Women's Secrets)—a book allegedly authored by the Catholic Bishop Albertus Magnus in 1478, but sometimes attributed to Henry of Saxony—found plenty to be disgusted about at both ends of a woman: "Women are so full of venom in their time of menstruation that they poison animals by their glare; they infect children in the cradle, they spot the cleanest mirror; and whenever men have sexual intercourse with them, they are made leprous and sometimes cancerous." Later, a Dr. des Laurens wrote: "How can this divine animal, full of reason and judgment, which we call man, be attracted by these obscene parts of woman, defiled with juices and located shamefully at the lowest part of the trunk?"[7]

Philosophical theories that pass judgment on women's reproductive organs or capacities without the least understanding of them tend to remind me of the argument that my friend overheard between her seven- and four-year-old sons and their five-year-old sister one morning while they were playing in their backyard. The boys were demonstrating how far each could pee, while their sister tried to show that she, too, could not only pee standing up, but that she could direct her stream. Finding herself with pee running down both thighs, she suddenly plopped herself down on the lawn and began sobbing, as her older brother solemnly pronounced his judgment in the deepest voice he could muster: "Ours is better."

As I have noted above, this juvenile "ours is better" kind of thinking emerged early in the writings that have powerfully influenced Eurocentric culture over the last 2,500 years or so. How interesting it is that even the writings of modern-day feminists have contained echoes of the recurrent theme of revulsion of the body—especially of the life-giving female body. For instance, Simone de Beauvoir (who never gave birth) expressed strong, negative feelings about birth in her influential book *The Second Sex*. She argued that giving birth is an act "that is not an activity in a human sense, and carries with it no pride in creation ... For she does not really make the baby, it makes itself within her; her flesh engenders flesh only, and she is quite incapable of establishing an existence that will have to establish itself." She goes on, "Ensnared by nature, the pregnant woman is plant and animal, a stockpile of colloids, an incubator, an egg; she scares children proud of their young straight bodies and makes young people titter contemptuously because she is a human being, a conscious and free individual, who has become life's passive instrument."[8] Apparently, for de Beauvoir, women must compete not only with men, but also with nature, which has the ability to "ensnare" them. Never in her writing did she express the view that it would be possible to live in harmony with men or with nature.

Shulamith Firestone, a generation after de Beauvoir, built on her predecessor's disgust of women's ability to give birth with the publication of her 1970 book *The Dialectic of Sex*. For Firestone, women's true adversary was biology, so the next logical step to free women from its "tyranny" was for the "underclass" of women to "seize control of reproduction." This meant "not only the full restoration to women of ownership of their own bodies, but also their (temporary) seizure of control of human fertility—the new population of biology as well as all the social institutions of child-bearing and child-rearing." Firestone never described how her envisioned revolution was to come about any more than Saint Augustine elaborated on what would have been a better design for women's bodies. Her faith in men's ability to control nature had no apparent limits ("Humanity has begun to transcend Nature"). "Soon," she wrote, "we shall have a complete understanding of the entire reproductive process in all its complexity, including the subtle dynamics of hormones and their full effects on the nervous system." Not only could we look forward to that happy day just around the corner, but this, too: "Several teams of scientists are working on the development of an artificial placenta. Even parthogenesis—virgin birth—could be developed very soon," she added hopefully.[9]

While Firestone was right that in vitro fertilization was just around the corner, she didn't know enough about biology to understand why that artificial placenta was unlikely to revolutionize pregnancy in the near future. Apparently lacking any knowledge of the history of midwifery, medicine, or birth, she argued strenuously for a reinforcement of the supremacy that the medical profession wielded over women's bodies. Although she clearly admired Mary Wollstonecraft, the first European woman to make a powerful call for human rights to be extended to women, she seemed to have missed what Wollstonecraft wrote after giving birth for the first time at the age of thirty-five (with a midwife), "Nothing could be more natural or easy than my labour."[10] She also missed (as did de Beauvoir) women's rights pioneer and philosopher Elizabeth Cady Stanton's statement after the birth of her sixth child:

> I never felt such sacredness in carrying a child as I have in the case of this one. She is the largest and most vigorous baby I have ever had, weighing twelve pounds. And yet my labor was short and easy. I laid down about fifteen minutes, and lone with my nurse and one female friend brought forth this big girl. I sat up immediately, changed my own clothes, put on a wet bandage, and, after a few hours' repose, sat up again. Am I not almost a savage? For what refined, delicate, genteel, civilized woman would get well in so indecently short a time?[11]

In that last sentence, Stanton was referring to the frequent observation made by nineteenth-century doctors that "savages" had easy births, whereas "civilized" women invariably had long, hard births. She, like the women in my community, had no feeling of inferiority to any other group of women when it came to the ability to give birth. In my opinion, her seven easy, unmedicated births undoubtedly were made possible by several factors: her well-documented reluctance to wear clothing that unduly restricted her movements or her ability to breathe as deeply as an active man, her awareness of the need for good nutrition, and her decision to hire a midwife instead of a doctor. A doctor in those days would likely have brought the chief tools and "medications" that doctors' bags almost invariably contained: a set of forceps, a scalpel for bloodletting, other metal instruments meant to extract babies whose lives were to be sacrificed so the mother's could be saved, some mercury chloride for purging, perhaps some leeches to help draw off more "excess" blood, and quinine for the induction of labor.

TWO MODELS OF MATERNITY CARE

The midwifery model recognizes that, as Professor G. J. Kloosterman pointed out, spontaneous labor in healthy women cannot be improved upon, and that the process of such labor is delicate enough that interference in the process may actually deflect it from its optimum course. Kloosterman knew, of course, that obstetricians were essential in the comparatively rare cases when pathological situations develop, but he cautioned that they should interfere only when necessary, in order not to *cause* complications in what otherwise would be a normal course of labor.

He was eloquent in his statements about the need for midwives to be an essential part of the maternity care team, and helped to bring about a system in the Netherlands in which women go directly to midwives for their maternity care. His assumption, of course, was that midwives would be the primary attendant at approximately three-quarters of all births and that they would, as they do in all western European countries, far outnumber obstetrician-gynecologists. These midwives are trained and trusted to know when to refer cases requiring consultation or referral to an obstetrician. This is just one way that the structure of the Dutch system protects women from unnecessary creation of pathology during the course of maternity care. In fact, if a Dutch woman wants to go straight to an obstetrician for her care, she must pay out of pocket for it. However, her midwifery care is covered by her national insurance, as is her obstetric care if her midwife deems it necessary.

About one-third of Dutch women choose to give birth in their homes. Dutch physicians and policy makers have long respected a woman's right to make this choice. (It should be said that some Dutch physicians wish to curb this right.) Another way the Dutch system displays its respect for midwifery knowledge is that its future obstetricians and gynecologists are exposed to normal births attended by midwives before they move into the necessary phase of their training that concentrates on pathology. This is one way that doctors in training can learn the many variations that can happen in normal labor and birth. It also has the effect of teaching them how well natural processes function when they are not disturbed and there is a calm atmosphere in the birth room. The end result is a doctor who knows when his interventions are unnecessary and understands that competent midwives are good at knowing when interventions are necessary. With this respect for and balance between the two essential professions for optimal maternity care—midwifery and obstetrics—the Dutch manage to provide a broad degree of maternal choice in place of birth and style of care without lowering safety standards. Their flexible system has produced some of the lowest morbidity and mortality rates in the world. One hopes they will be able to maintain it in the years to come.

Professor Kloosterman's intellectual forefather was Hendrik van

Deventer, a Dutch physician-author who published a much-translated textbook for midwives and male midwives in the early eighteenth century. Van Deventer, who was married to a midwife, set an early tone of respect in the Netherlands for midwives and for women's innate ability to give birth. At the same time, he recognized that many midwives of his time needed better training and proposed that a midwifery school should be established in every city. A great believer in natural childbirth, he believed that obstetricians should only become involved in the presence of clear pathology. He rarely used instruments and appreciated how much upright postures facilitated birth. He wrote: "Infants by their own gravity pass betwixt the bones into the neck of the womb, which is easily dilated by the force of pressing pains..." About induction, he remarked, "I know, indeed, that medicines are of much force to stir up pains; but a great many observations have taught me that very strong forcing medicines have done a great deal of harm to women in labour."[12]

US MATERNITY CARE MOVES EARLY INTO UNCHARTED TERRITORY

US doctors with the kind of appreciation for women's innate ability to give birth and for the necessity of midwives expressed by van Deventer and Kloosterman have existed, but sadly, their influence has not lived after them. As for US midwives, the careers of those who worked during the early colonial period were mostly celebrated in their epitaphs or by their families or communities. None wrote a book. Mrs. Thomas Whitemore, of Marlboro, Vermont, was reported never to have lost a woman in the course of attending about two thousand births.[13] A Long Island midwife, who attended the births of 1,300 babies between 1745 and 1774, was said to have lost only two babies and no mothers. Remember, no one was performing C-sections on live women in those times, and midwives didn't own or use forceps. Historians Wertz and Wertz wrote, "... we know that

[US] midwives caused no recorded epidemics of puerperal fever among their patients," and mentioned as well that a "distinguished medical historian of Virginia has calculated that the illiterate black midwives of that state spread less infection than did doctors until the end of the 19th century."[14] Even so, the few voices of doctors who understood the value of midwives were eventually drowned out by those who saw midwives as competitors for fees they thought should be theirs. As I mentioned earlier, Dr. Hugh L. Hodge's idea, with his 1838 publication, was to establish what he called "the universal practice of obstetrics" by scaring women into accepting doctors in place of midwives. Practically speaking, this effort was aimed at keeping women from having any power of decision in matters of childbirth.

I have always found it interesting that even though midwives were well represented among the victims who were persecuted and executed during the great European witch hunt that raged from about 1450 until 1750, resulting in the deaths of, at the very least, 120,000 people (mostly women and a large number of them midwives), the thought of stopping the profession of midwifery itself seems never to have occurred to European medical men.[15] The fact that midwives from several countries had written textbooks during the seventeenth and eighteenth centuries and that they enjoyed the support of some of the royal families is perhaps a partial explanation for why midwifery survived in Europe during the period when it was being annihilated in North America. The most decisive phase in the medical campaign in the US to eliminate the midwife lasted from about 1900 to 1930. In that campaign, certain influential doctors portrayed the midwife as a "relic of the barbaric past," as un-American, cruel, ignorant, incapable of learning, and filthy, making the most of racist and anti-immigrant sentiments that were easy to exploit in a country that had only put the institution of slavery aside a few decades earlier and had been accepting huge waves of immigrants. In fact, many of the European immigrant midwives had received excellent educations in midwifery schools in their respective countries before their arrival here. Public health departments existed mostly in cities and rarely bothered to assess the outcomes of the rural midwives of all colors who were working throughout the US at that time. Instead, large amounts of antimidwife propaganda articles were published in popular women's magazines. One such article appeared in *Harper's Magazine* in 1930, with its nurse-author declaring: "Rat-pie midwifery may often be picturesque to the student of folklore, but what a commentary upon our national public health is its continued existence in this twentieth century!" At no point in her article did she explain why she chose the term "rat-pie" to describe midwifery, but her intent to evoke disgust in her readers is obvious.[16] Such articles didn't mention that many of these "barbaric" midwives had graduated from midwifery schools that still existed in the US during the early twentieth century, or that maternal death rates actually rose when US women began giving birth in hospitals in large numbers. Epidemics of childbed fever were common in hospitals right through the twenties, despite careful aseptic and antiseptic techniques.[17] The same disease, however, was rare among women who were attended by their rural midwives, who generally learned from the elder midwives with whom they apprenticed not to put their fingers or hands into the women's vaginas. The granny midwives of the US South had actually enjoyed high cultural autonomy and prestige within the slave economy in which black women were breeders. Not only did they bestow healing among the enslaved women, they attended a significant number of white births, including those of the plantation owners' wives.[18] All of this history was forgotten during the antimidwife propaganda campaign.

It wasn't until the early twentieth century that the legal right of women to serve as midwives began to be questioned in some states. (It should be noted that it was only men who had a part in making laws during this period.) In many states, midwifery was protected to a small degree by statutes that declared that midwifery was not the practice of medicine. However, in Massachusetts, under the Birth Registration Act of 1897, doctors or midwives were supposed to register births, but only doctors could be licensed to practice, and in 1907 the Massachusetts Supreme Court ruled that midwifery and obstetrics were synonymous. If a midwife complied with the registration law, she automatically admitted that she was violating the Medical Practice Act. Hanna Porn, a hardworking Finnish American midwife who served the Finnish and Swedish communities in Gardner, Massachusetts, was tried ten times between 1905 and 1908. Each time, an all-male jury convicted her, and it didn't matter that the four doctors who testified against her had a neonatal mortality rate almost double hers for the year prior to her court case, or that she charged her clients about a third of what they did.[19]

Black midwives and white midwives who lived in rural areas usually learned by apprenticeship with an elder midwife or from their experiences tending to their farm animals. My own great-grandmother, Lois Butler Middleton, who worked as a rural midwife in Iowa between approximately 1870 and 1903, surely got much of her knowledge from the culture in which she lived, with the many chances that rural children had to observe nature's workings. I learned from a family diary that my great-grandfather had opinions about what could happen when people get too alienated from nature. "Town children are not as brave or smart as country children," he said. "They are too timid." I learned a little about what he meant upon listening to a story from one of my older neighbors when my husband and I first settled in rural Tennessee. Mrs. Smith, who had given birth at home to premature twins during the forties, told me about how the doctor (possibly a "town child") who was attending their birth closed up his bag, said, "They'll never make it," and abruptly left. At that point, her mother, who had been in the kitchen, had the oven ready to serve as an incubator for the tiny girls, just as she and countless other farm wives had been accustomed to do with runt pigs. "You never saw such big strapping girls as those two turned out to be!" Mrs. Smith told me.

When it comes to maternity care in the US, appearances often count more than reality. For instance, the argument that childbirth was far too dangerous for midwives to be trusted to recognize complications that might develop (this was one of the most repeated assertions during the antimidwife campaign) directly contradicted the reality that the replacements for the midwife—the newly created obstetric nurses—were expected to do just that. However, because these nurses were often harshly scolded if a baby arrived before the doctor, they often resorted to holding women's legs together to prevent birth, a dangerous practice that can result in neurological damage to the babies. A real midwife would never hold a woman's legs together to prevent birth.

BRUTAL, IGNORANT PRACTICES BECOME THE NORM FOR A MAJORITY OF US WOMEN

When there are no midwives in a position to question the extremes that can come from a strictly medical (illness) model of birth, irrational and even cruel routines can quickly replace common sense and justifiable practice. It can be hard for us in the US to fully appreciate how surprised Western European midwives and doctors are to learn how extremely invasive and rough US obstetric practice was compared to the European norm around the time when birth moved into hospitals in the early twentieth century—that forceps could have been used so liberally, so automatically, even in those cases when the baby would have fallen out if nature had taken its course. Doctors and midwives in no other country would have found forceps rates of 65 to 70 percent of all births acceptable or imaginable.

At the same time, some thoughtful doctors understood the temptations that forceps could present to their colleagues. William Hunter, an eighteenth-century Scottish anatomist and leading obstetrician of his time, for instance, wrote that he thought that forceps had done more harm than good. He would show his students how rusty his forceps were from disuse and say that it was a shame that they had ever been invented, for "where they save one they murder twenty."[20] An eighteenth-century English obstetrician, James Blundell, addressed his colleagues in a book published in 1834:

> I strenuously dissuade you from making familiar companions of your instruments because they are not wanted ... The very fact that an *accoucheur* [obstetrician], on all occasions, puts the lever into his pocket when he goes to attend a labor, proves that he is an officious, a meddlesome, and therefore, to my mind, a bad *accoucheur.* Some men seem to have a sort of instinctive impulse to put the lever or forceps into the vagina. "Lead yourselves not into temptation"; if you put your instruments into your pocket, they are very apt to slip out of your pocket into the uterus. Patience and good nature, are two useful obstetric instruments which may be fearlessly carried to every labor.[21]

These voices of reason within the British medical profession regarding the use of forceps surely had some good effect in curtailing their unnecessary use. It is also worth noting that the midwifery profession was sufficiently established and healthy in every European country, such that midwives far outnumbered physicians doing obstetrics. European midwives were involved in the training of doctors and thus were usually able to keep the use of forceps to a minimum. In contrast, no midwives were allowed to work in US hospitals when large numbers of women began giving birth there. Most doctors weren't about to sit with women during labor, so the profession of the obstetric nurse was created to do the work of the midwife up to a few minutes before birth—but without the voice, training, and status of a midwife. The nurse's job was to make sure that the doctor arrived before the baby did and to stand aside when he arrived. Hugh L. Hodge would have been pleased at how thoroughly his successors carried out his idea of teaching women to fear birth, because US women obediently filed into hospitals for decades with no idea that a fuller set of options and better care existed elsewhere.

My own collection of medical textbooks includes one published in the US in 1895 that was among the first to include photographs of birth. Because doctors at that time weren't required to attend classes, this book would have been the first introduction to what birth looked like for many medical apprentices. The photo of a "normal birth" features a woman lying flat on her back, her legs apart and strapped in stirrups, so thoroughly draped that only her bottom is visible. Five gowned men who appear to be in their thirties surround her, as one conducts the "delivery." All four fingers of the doctor's right hand are inside the woman's anus as her baby's head emerges. According to the accompanying text, this was a demonstration of the "correct" way to keep the mother from injuring herself as she births her baby. The last photos of the series show the doctor pushing hard on the woman's abdomen to manually force delivery of the placenta, a measure that the author writes is necessary to prevent the woman from bleeding too much. However, the visible blood loss considered in this textbook to be normal was enough to be counted as a serious hemorrhage today.[22] In fact, impatient and forcible removal of the placenta is more likely to cause hemorrhage than to prevent it.

Many experienced doctors in 1895 would not have considered large blood loss especially dangerous, since "heroic bloodletting" was actually recommended for a long list of conditions during pregnancy and labor. Many nineteenth-century medical textbooks were written with an assumption that pregnant women often suffered from having too much blood (they weren't having periods, after all), so regular blood removal was necessary to maintain good health.

"Women without evidence of specific disease were bled as often as 6 or 8 times during the latter months; and many cases are recorded in which the depletions were performed every fortnight as a routine, or as many as 50 to 90 times in the course of a pregnancy when symptoms were pronounced."[23] Bloodletting was even used to stop hemorrhaging, following the "logic" that losing even more blood would produce blood clotting and stop the hemorrhage. One doctor wrote in the mid-nineteenth century:

> The officiousness of nurses and friends very often thwarts the best-directed measure of the physician, by an overweening desire to make the patient "comfortable" . . . all this should be strictly forbidden. Conversation should be prohibited the patient . . . Nothing is more common than for the patient's friends to object to [bloodletting], urging as a reason, that "she has lost blood enough." Of this they are in no respect suitable judges.[24]

It was the end of the nineteenth century before bloodletting was given up as a treatment by US doctors. The odd thing is that it was more likely to be done to middle class women than to poor women (who would have been attended by midwives), because men of means were easy to hoodwink into the idea that the more expensive style of care was superior. I wish that medical students were taught more about the history of their own profession, since knowledge of history can teach caution in introducing new, untried techniques and "medications."

How little many US doctors themselves knew about labor and birth during the early twentieth century is evident from a 1912 study of obstetric education in 120 medical schools carried out by J. Whitridge Williams, an influential textbook author whose book, *Willliams Obstetrics*, is in its twenty-third edition at the time of this writing. This scathing report found an "appallingly slight experience which many had before being appointed to professorships." Of his own institution, Johns Hopkins, Williams wrote, "I would unhesitatingly state that my own students are unfit on graduation to practice obstetrics in its broad sense, and are scarcely prepared to handle normal cases."[25] Historian Judith Walzer Leavitt wrote, "Williams found that most medical students had the opportunity during their training to watch only one woman deliver, and one quarter of the medical schools admitted that their graduates were not competent to practice obstetrics,"[26] and there are historical records of doctors who were expected to pose as competent practitioners when they had never witnessed a birth of any kind.

The solution that many doctors then promoted was to join the campaign to eliminate midwives in order to create unlimited opportunities for doctors to upgrade their knowledge and experience. Physicians were able to access the power of the state through their professional organizations, and to control licensing legislation that would either limit the midwives' sphere of activity or to entirely stop their practice. For the first time, poor and immigrant women were brought into hospitals for care (DeLee actually paid them to come to his hospital in Chicago). This was a time before aseptic technique was practiced, before antibiotics were introduced, and before modern surgical techniques had been developed. Maternal and infant mortality both rose during the first decade of the twentieth century in Washington DC, New York, New Jersey, and Boston as doctors attended more births, midwives attended fewer, and more women entered hospitals to give birth.[27] The poor outcomes, however, did nothing to stem the rapidly increasing rate of hospital births, because they received no publicity. This shameful pattern of hiding poor outcomes continues to this day in the US, as I will explain later in this book.

My more ancient medical book collection contains two excellent works published in the US that apparently received less attention than they should have. The first is George Engelmann's *Labor Among Primitive Peoples*, which I have already mentioned, published in 1882. Engelmann, a founding member of the American Gynecological Society and professor of gynecology at the St. Louis Postgraduate School of Medicine, filled his book with excellent drawings of indigenous women from many parts of the world, nude and in labor, surrounded by their attendants. In each case, the artist clearly saw the beauty in each woman, the power and the grace in how she positioned herself to give birth. Engelmann introduced his book with a comment that he understood that his colleagues would regard a comparison of the "crude methods" of primitive peoples and peoples of former civilizations with the teachings of the scientific obstetrics of his time as "amusing and interesting," but a few pages later commented on how reasonable some of their practices seemed to him:

> A vast and important fund of knowledge may be derived from a study of the various positions occupied by women of different peoples in their labors. According to their build, to the shape of the pelvis, they stand, squat, kneel or lie upon the belly; so also they vary their position in various stages of labor according to the position of the child's head in the pelvis. Does the great number of natural labors resulting not point to a law greatly at variance with the teachings of modern obstetrics? Is it not evident that different positions should be given in stages of labor, and in its various periods?

He added:

> The savage mother, the Negress, the Australian or
> Indian, still governed by her instinct, is far in advance
> of the ordinary woman of our civilization.[28]

How exciting it was for me to find Engelmann's book and to
understand how an open-minded, observant US obstetrician of the
late nineteenth century tried to impart some of the midwifery
model of care to his colleagues and students.[29] If only they had
wished to learn from him.

The second work was written by Alice Stockham, an obstetrician-gynecologist who was a contemporary of Engelmann, and the
fifth US woman to become a doctor. A friend of Leo Tolstoy and
Havelock Ellis, she advocated for women in many ways, including
dress and dietary reform, birth control, gender equality, and male
and female sexual fulfillment in marriage. Her book, *Tokology*,
published in 1891, contains advice that is still as good as it was then.
"Motion is a Law of Nature. All animal life is full of activity.
Remaining quietly in closely heated rooms frequently causes disease in the pregnant woman . . . Going up stairs is the best way to
get desired exercise in a short time." Stockham favored warm, deep
baths as a way to favor relaxation during labor, along with massage,
and many changes of position during the course of labor. On tightly
laced corsets, the fashion no decent woman was supposed to do
without, she answered a group of critics, who asked: "Does she not
need a corset? What if one cannot hold herself up without a corset?
Will she wear a corset under or over the princess waist? Does a loose
corset do any harm? . . . And faster and faster the questions come,
until my ears are deafened with corset! Corset! Corset! . . . if women
had common sense, instead of fashion sense, the corset would not
exist," she declared.[30]

THE IMPACT OF THE TWILIGHT SLEEP ERA

If more leading doctors had taken George Engelmann's book seriously and more influential women had followed the advice in Alice Stockham's book, it's possible that the twilight sleep era could have been avoided. As it happened, though, during World War I, many prominent women took an active part in promoting "twilight sleep" as the best anesthesia that could be imagined. Because there had been a number of well-publicized maternal deaths caused by chloroform and ether, women were afraid of these older kinds of anesthesia but trusted science and medicine to come up with something better. Unfortunately, they fell for a nice advertising phrase. Twilight sleep consisted of an injection of morphine, followed by scopolamine, an amnesiac. Once the morphine wore off, the pain was back, and the woman was left alone with it. Terror-stricken and lacking their normal social inhibitions because of the effects of the scopolamine, the laboring women shrieked and cursed so loudly and thrashed around so violently that nurses were instructed to routinely strap them to their beds during labor or put them in special cages and to put plugs in the laboring women's ears. This practice only came to an end when the natural childbirth movement finally succeeded in pressuring maternity wards to allow fathers to be present throughout labor and for the births of their babies during the seventies. Such overt cruelty did not go down well when fathers were present. But it wasn't just the relaxation of the prohibition against fathers being present at births that spelled the end of the twilight sleep era; it was the advent of the increasingly routine use of the epidural that pushed twilight sleep out of the picture once and for all.

By the sixties, even though twilight sleep was no longer the medication of choice in the hospital where I gave birth, many obstetricians were still tying women down when the time came to push the baby out. It was a rude surprise to learn, only while they were doing it to you, deep in labor, that it had been their plan all along to shackle you to the delivery table before they cut your perineum, inserted the forceps, dragged out your baby, and then carried her away. The care was so obviously crazy to me and countless others that the time was ripe for a reform movement.

WOMEN'S COMPLAINTS SURFACE IN
THE *LADIES' HOME JOURNAL*

In 1958, the *Ladies' Home Journal*, a popular women's magazine, published a letter from a registered nurse who remained anonymous for fear of reprisal. Her letter complained of cruelty and dangerous practices she had witnessed in maternity wards. In response, letters poured in from all parts of the country and were published over the next several months in the magazine. Some excerpts:

> With leather cuffs strapped around my wrists and legs, I was left alone for nearly eight hours until the actual delivery.

> My obstetrician wanted to get home for dinner. When I was taken to the delivery room my legs were tied way up in the air and spread as far apart as they would go . . . when I was securely tied down I was left alone.

> What about the nameless parade of "interns" who appear unannounced, probe our trapped bodies and "scan" our progress? . . . Since my husband is a veterinarian, I happen to know that even animal maternity cases are treated with a little more grace than is accorded human mothers.[31]

> The doctor . . . went out to make a house call. One hour later my legs were released in the stirrups and held

together by a nurse who sat on my knees, up on the delivery table, mind you, because the baby was coming so fast.

I was strapped on the delivery table. My doctor had not arrived and the nurses held my legs together. I was helpless and at their mercy. They held my baby back until the doctor came into the room.[32]

The exposé of maternity ward abuse helped to push along a new trend that began in the US in the twentieth century, an attempt to resuscitate the midwifery profession after a long period of cultural amnesia. A midwifery pioneer named Mary Breckinridge, daughter of the US minister to Russia during Grover Cleveland's administration, had already begun an ambitious project to provide midwifery services to women in the doctorless, remote mountains of eastern Kentucky in 1925. I say "ambitious" because this service eventually covered an area of about one thousand square miles that was accessible only by horseback, with few roads or trails but many rivers and creeks to ford and ridgetops where footing was treacherous even in the best weather conditions. Breckinridge thought the people there needed both nursing and midwifery, so she recruited two British nurse-midwives to help her start what she called the Frontier Nursing Service (FNS). (Note that she elected not to use the "bad" word "midwifery.") Breckinridge set a model of keeping careful records of all of the births the midwives attended, a model that was followed by many other midwifery services that were to follow hers. For forty years until her death in 1965, this maternity service, which was predominantly a home birth practice for its first thirty years, produced some of the best birth outcomes in the US, with a lower maternal death rate than was being achieved in urban hospitals during the same period.

Despite the impressive statistics of the FNS and other services such as the Lobenstine Midwifery Clinic in Harlem and the Catholic Maternity Institute in Santa Fe, New Mexico, acceptance of the nurse-midwives by obstetricians came slowly and incompletely, as many, following the advice presented by Dr. Hugh L. Hodge, continued to view midwives as competitors instead of necessary members of the same team. By the end of the first decade of the twenty-first century, only 8 percent of US births were being attended by nurse-midwives, with a mere 0.5 percent attended by certified professional midwives (CPMs), a more recent arrival on the scene. It has taken a monumental amount of work for all kinds of midwives to gain legal recognition, a state at a time, usually against medical opposition that often worked to maintain the status quo: "No midwives wanted here."

Nurse-midwives have found support from some obstetricians, including author Harold Speert, who optimistically commented in his *Obstetrics and Gynecology in America: A History*, published in 1980, "Nurse-midwives and their assistants have thus helped rectify what many obstetric authorities have considered the greatest weakness in American obstetrics, a lack of emotional support of the parturient in pregnancy and labor."[33] In hindsight, he should have specified "for a small segment of US women." If the leadership of the American College (now changed to "Congress") of Obstetricians and Gynecologists (ACOG) had felt then as Harold Speert apparently did, it's possible that today we could be approaching a time when more than two-thirds of US laboring women have a midwife in attendance, instead of a mere 8.5 percent.

Sadly for US women and babies, the policies that have been adopted by ACOG ever since the first national midwifery organization, the American College of Nurse-Midwives (ACNM), was established in 1955 have continued to reinforce the dominance that ACOG established over ACNM from the beginning. In order for the ACNM to exist, its leaders had to agree to a joint statement of practice relationships that provided for an "interdependence" between obstetricians and midwives that was "lopsided, that is, not mutual, and thus not real interdependence," according to past president of ACNM, Judith P. Rooks.[34] For the most part, this has meant that nurse-midwifery has been allowed to exist only when no obstetrician in a particular geographical area strongly objects. As for obstetricians themselves, even being known as a midwife-friendly obstetrician can be hard on one's career or professional relationships.

I first became aware of how strongly some obstetricians oppose the establishment of nurse-midwifery practices in 1980 when Congressman Albert Gore Jr. held hearings on the obstacles two nurse-midwives faced in Nashville, Tennessee. The midwives were denied the right to open an independent practice, even though they had arranged for emergency backup from an obstetrician. These midwives, like Mary Breckinridge, had been providing care to poor women, but that didn't matter (though the midwives had thought it would). They were surprised to be denied access to every hospital in the city when they sought such privileges.[35] Even after the hearings, their practice was denied. The obstetrician who had originally proposed to work with them was quickly pressured by colleagues to renege, to the point that he left town and never returned. Such a display of where the power truly lies is unforgettable and disheartening. One of those midwives never again worked as a midwife and turned instead to nursing. As for me, I noticed how little it mattered that the two nurse-midwives had a legal right to practice midwifery in Tennessee; their licenses appeared to be almost meaningless.

Longstanding midwifery services can still be closed down on short notice, despite their popularity and the number of women who prefer midwifery care. Sometimes nurse-midwives who have been working for fifteen years or more find themselves out of a job overnight and unable to find another midwifery position in their city. In 2010, a popular nurse-midwifery service in Ventura County, California, was forced to close by the chief executive officer of the area's community hospital, who claimed without offering any evidence that having a neonatal intensive care unit (NICU) had suddenly become necessary if a hospital was to allow nurse-midwives to continue having admitting and discharge privileges for the low-risk women in their practice. (The hospital had a maternity service and nursery but no NICU.) The CEO never explained why the doctors who attended the births of high-risk women (who would presumably give birth more often than low-risk women to babies with complications) were able to function without one.[36]

What is rarely recognized in US mainstream culture is that countries which routinely turn out better maternity care results than the US (at much lower cost) all have the power to determine how many midwives and how many physicians will be part of their maternity care system. In none of these countries are midwives denied the ability to be lead professionals in hospitals, with admitting and discharging privileges. Contrast this situation with the difficulty we have in the US to keep even a relatively small number of birth centers open, despite their popularity and documented good results. Even longstanding midwifery services in hospitals in some cities can be closed on short notice, despite the protests of the women who prefer or have booked midwifery care. Consider, too, the obstacles faced by women who live in smaller cities, towns, and rural areas who wish to gain access to the services of a midwife.

The question of home birth raises the ante even higher than does the question of an autonomous midwifery profession. Even though the American Public Health Association, the Royal College of Obstetricians and Gynaecologists (RCOG) in the UK, and several Canadian medical societies approve of planned home birth as a safe option for women with low-risk pregnancies, ACOG continues to oppose it to the same degree it did in the seventies, when one of its presidents claimed that home birth was a form of "child abuse." Today, their favorite slogan is that home delivery should be only for pizza. Midwifery—whether we are discussing certified professional midwives, certified nurse-midwives, or certified midwives (the three designations of midwives currently licensed to work in the US)—is still far from being a core component of maternity care.

In 2010, women who live in New York City suddenly lost their right to have a home birth with a midwife legally attending them, a right that a growing number had been choosing in recent years. This restriction of options occurred because of the bankruptcy of the only hospital in the city with maternity care policies progressive enough to open its doors to clients choosing home birth (who might require transfer to a hospital during or after labor). The city's thirteen nurse-midwives (the only midwives legally permitted to attend home births there) were all obliged under state law to be approved by a hospital or obstetrician, in addition to their professional training, certification, and state licensure.[37] This time, however, the mothers who wanted these midwives to be freed from these unreasonable strictures managed to put enough pressure on the state legislature to pass a new law freeing the midwives from the yoke that ACOG had lobbied so hard to keep in place.

SMOKE AND MIRRORS

The scientific research enterprise, like other human activities, is built on a foundation of trust. Scientists trust that the results reported by others are valid. Society trusts that the results of research reflect an honest attempt by scientists to describe the world accurately and without bias. The level of trust that has characterized science and its relationship with society has contributed to a period of unparalleled scientific productivity. But this trust will endure only if the scientific community devotes itself to exemplifying and transmitting the values associated with ethical scientific conduct.

—National Academy of Engineering and Institute of Medicine, *On Being a Scientist*

Judging by its public statements and actions since 1955, ACOG can be counted on to resist most attempts to make midwives available to a larger segment of the public or to provide women with choices regarding place of birth. Since the seventies, ACOG has issued public statements depicting home birth as a selfish and dangerous choice for women to make, ignoring the many well-designed studies that have indicated the contrary. During the same period, several US medical journals found the space to print articles that I would call propaganda—the use of words and numbers to push forward a specific agenda—and not genuine scientific inquiry. In other words, what was presented as "science" actually involved invalid conclusions based on data that was manipulated to support a viewpoint that the data, upon proper analysis, did not support. It would require a much bigger book than this one for me to include an exhaustive list and discussion of these articles, but I'll mention a sampling that illustrate some of the statistical and deliberately deceptive tricks that have been used.

A good one to start with is the February 1983 issue of the *Southern Medical Journal*, which included an article with the title: "Home Birth: Negative Implications Derived from a Hospital-based Birthing Suite." The article's five doctor-authors sought to determine if pregnant women could be screened accurately enough to identify those who would be safe candidates for home birth and those who would not. Using a hospital room that was labeled a birthing suite as their "simulated home birth," they first chose a group of 440 women they judged to be at low risk for birth complications. After 38 of the women decided against participation and 12 decided to have real home births, the doctors were left with 390. Of the 390, the doctors found that only 41 percent of the women they had guessed would be low risk were able to give birth in the hospital "simulated home birth" room. Of course, the chief defects of the study were that it involved no actual home births, no experienced midwives, and no competent home birth doctors.[38]

Another pseudoscientific study published in the *American Journal of Obstetrics and Gynecology* in the early eighties and authored by two Dutch obstetricians claimed to give "more or less definite evidence that the obstetric system prevailing in the Netherlands is not adequate from the point of view of neonatal morbidity." Neonatal morbidity (newborn trauma) can be defined in many ways, but most of the data used in this study related to blood gas analysis of cord blood (which can, when properly done, be one indication among many as to whether a baby is in trouble or not). The charge of inadequacy of the Dutch obstetric system made by obstetricians from a country in which nearly 40 percent of all births were home births was apparently too tempting for the journal's editors to resist, no matter how poor its design. The authors of the study based their conclusion on the outcomes of eighty-five midwife-assisted home births compared with twenty-seven hospital births conducted by doctors all in one city (an absurdly small sample). There was a large difference between the two groups, with the cord blood values of the midwives' babies being less favorable than the doctors' babies.[39] These data were interpreted by the authors to mean that babies born in hospitals with obstetricians in charge instead of midwives were less likely to be neurologically damaged by the birth process than those born at home under the care of midwives.

Three widely respected Dutch obstetricians, Drs. Treffers, van Alten, and Pel, then wrote a letter to the journal's editor criticizing both the methodology of the study as well as its sweeping conclusions. No Dutch medical journal would have accepted the report because of its flaws, and the authors' study had never been presented to Dutch colleagues (who would have found it laughable). "References were made to several articles and these not accessible to the English-reading public because the publications are written in Dutch," the study's critics pointed out, adding that "this investigation seems to be rather inadequate to warrant the far-reaching conclusions about an obstetric system that covers 180,000 births per year." They went on to explain why the cord values of the two groups were so different. Whereas the obstetricians cut the cords immediately after birth and sent the samples to the lab for analysis, the midwives' usual practice was to clamp the cord much later and store the sample at room temperature for quite a while before they could get it to a lab. These factors alone were enough to account for the difference in cord blood values between the two groups and had nothing at all to do with the relative well-being of the babies in either group.[40] A lot of ink was wasted on the Dutch "study," which revealed nothing more than the clear editorial bias of the US journal against midwifery and home birth and the irritation of the article's authors, who complained, "In the Netherlands the midwives operate as totally free and independent agents, not subjected to any supervising authority."[41]

A method that some US obstetricians have used in attempts to discredit home birth has been to publish studies that base their conclusions on comparisons between planned hospital births and planned home births, while relying solely on information drawn from birth certificates. This renders the data invalid, since the "planned home birth" data derived from birth certificates commonly include lots of births that weren't really planned to be at home-premature births that happened in a vehicle on the way to a hospital, births following pregnancies in which there was no prenatal care, involuntary home births by mothers in poor health, unassisted births by unmarried teen moms too shocked to know how to assist a baby to breathe, or even births by women who didn't realize they were pregnant.[42] Such was the method chosen for a highly misleading and much discredited study (known as the "Pang study") published by another major US obstetrics journal in 2002. You guessed it—it found an increased risk with home birth.[43] In 2010 a study comparing planned home birth with planned hospital birth was published in the *American Journal of Obstetrics & Gynecology* (AJOG)—a meta-analysis that I'll call the "Wax study."[44] Meta-analysis is simply a way of gathering together several smaller studies of a given subject and examining them collectively if one needs a larger number of cases in an area of research in which almost every study is small and randomization is impossible (as in home birth). Since results of meta-analyses can be manipulated according to which studies are included and which are not, much obviously depends upon the criteria chosen for inclusion and also on how each measured outcome is reviewed. In addition, the validity of meta-analysis depends upon consistency and clarity of methodology, so each meta-analysis should clearly state its own rules at the outset and then follow them. Explanation of methodology should be clear enough to eliminate guesswork as to how numbers are counted. Additionally, it's important that researchers then present only those conclusions that can be supported by the data presented. If not, meta-analysis can easily descend into the realm of propaganda, far from the locus of scientific inquiry where it should keep itself.

The Wax study rather quickly suggests its bias, for by the time one reads the third sentence of its seven pages, its credibility is hurt by the irrelevant repetition of the position of the American Congress of Obstetricians and Gynecologists—that ACOG "does not support home birth, citing safety concerns and lack of rigorous scientific study."[45] ACOG's concerns about safety ring hollow, given the lack of evidence that home birth for low-risk women is dangerous when assisted by qualified midwives or doctors. Furthermore, it seems valid to question why the organization centers its concerns around *planned* home birth (which involves less than 1 percent of US births) and not on the rising (and underreported) maternal death rate, a problem with much wider implications that I discuss in the following chapter.

The title of the Wax study specifies "*planned* home birth vs. *planned* hospital births" (emphasis mine), and yet it includes without reservation the already discredited Pang study—the very one that lost its claim to validity because of the unplanned home births that it admittedly included.

Such fundamental defects notwithstanding, *AJOG* then extended the reach of the Wax study by initially releasing it as "An Article in Press," accompanied by a press release to both international medical journals and regular media months before its actual print publication date. This approach was heavy on fanfare but light on careful presentation of valid science, because most reporters probably thought it unnecessary (as well as inconvenient) to read the article in full and so depended instead on trusting the validity of the information included in the abstract and press release of a peer-reviewed journal. The Wax study quickly received press coverage in most English-speaking countries. Mentioned early were maternal outcomes after planned home births, including perineal lacerations, hemorrhage, and infections, all of which were significantly lower in the planned home births than in the planned hospital births. However, the significance of the prevention of these sometimes major problems was effectively diminished by its juxtaposition to the main (and much contested) conclusion of the Wax study—that planned home births showed two to three times higher neonatal mortality rates than planned hospital births. By making the unwarranted assumption that babies' interests were opposed to those of the mother (a false assumption for which the authors presented no credible evidence), they created the stepping stone for the most overreaching leap of all—"less medical intervention during planned home birth is associated with a tripling of neonatal mortality." Such a conclusion may fit a widely held myth, but ethical science does not seek to create or reinforce myths. Nevertheless, this, the weakest part of the study, made sensationalistic, international headlines.

Soon after its online release, the Wax study's press release elicited an almost worshipful editorial from *The Lancet*, a widely read British medical journal, which accepted the main conclusion of the study without question when it stated: "A recent meta-analysis published in the *American Journal of Obstetrics & Gynecology* provides the strongest evidence so far that home birth can, after all, be harmful to newborn babies."[46] The problem is that the study did no such thing. It's relevant first to understand that perinatal mortality, as defined by the Wax study, consisted of all stillbirths after twenty weeks of gestation or weighing at least five hundred grams plus the deaths of live-born babies within the first twenty-eight days after birth; and neonatal mortality consisted of the deaths of live-born babies within the first twenty-eight days after birth. In other words, neonatal mortality was defined as a *subset* of perinatal mortality. We have to wonder then how the authors of the Wax study managed to find a much higher death rate in the subset of neonatal mortality than in the larger set of perinatal mortality in both planned home births and hospital births. Incredibly, they ask us to believe that this impossible result could be true.

In fact, five of the authors whose studies were included in the Wax study's meta-analysis found so many numerical, statistical, and logical errors in the Wax paper that they signed a letter to the *AJOG* editor nearly as long as the Wax study itself, detailing a host of serious errors.[47] All felt that their data had been misused. An especially egregious flaw was that the Dutch study that yielded 88 percent of the nearly half a million total births considered in the Wax study was only used in considering two specific outcomes, neither of which was the main conclusion, the supposedly off-the-charts neonatal mortality rate.[48] On the other hand, the discredited Pang study, which alone provided more than half of the neonatal deaths but just one-third of the births, *was* tabulated for neonatal mortality. Valid? Hardly.

Besides the failure to adhere to its own stated rules about limiting the meta-analysis to births planned for home or hospital by including the Pang study, the Wax study's final choice of twelve published studies featured certain oddities as to its criteria for inclusion. For example, the Wax study included a study involving only eleven births[49] while omitting a much larger study (about five thousand births) that was methodologically sound, for reasons one can only guess at.[50]

Then there was the claim made by the authors of the Wax study that planned home births were characterized by a greater proportion of neonatal deaths attributed to respiratory distress and failed resuscitation. Once again, the Wax study failed to present credible data to support this conclusion; four of the twelve primary articles chosen for the meta-analysis did not support this conclusion. One study reported not a single death that was attributed to respiratory distress or failed resuscitation in the home birth group.[51] In another, one of two home birth fatalities was attributed to asphyxia, while four of seven in the hospital group listed asphyxia as the cause of death.[52] A third article reported one death of an infant who had no onset of spontaneous respiration; in this paper, the hospital birth comparison group consisted of only sixty-seven births, with no asphyxiation deaths reported.[53] The critics of the Wax study remarked that it remains a mystery as to how these three articles could be interpreted to support the claim made. As the *Lancet* reported in November 2010:

> Their 9-page letter points to mistakes in definitions, numerical errors, selective and mistaken inclusion and exclusion of studies, conflation of association and causation, and additional statistical problems. The result is a paper that is 'nonsensical.' They ask that the editors of *AJOG* act with 'urgency and concern' to address the 'insupportable conclusion' of the article. Their letter is dated Sep 15, 2010. So far, the editors of [*AJOG*] have yet to respond in public.[54]

The letter demanded that the journal publish a full retraction of the paper and send out an "equally well-disseminated press release" announcing the retraction. Academics all, they commented on how misleading it was for the press release to advertise that data from about 500,000 births were extracted for the study to support the reliability of the neonatal death rates mentioned above, when the text of the study (not the press release nor abstract) actually stated that the neonatal death rates were drawn from only 50,000 births. In other words, the Wax study attempted to fluff its credibility by inclusion of the large amount of births in the Dutch study but then ignored it in the tabulation of results related to neonatal mortality (the one outcome that the authors obviously considered their most important finding). The Wax study's critics further remarked that their own studies accounted for more than 93 percent of the 549,607 births considered in the Wax paper and pointed out that its flaws were systemic—far too deep for typographical errors to be corrected or for certain statistics to be recalculated and presented as corrections in a future edition of the journal. Rather, they urged *AJOG*'s senior editorial staff to examine the process that allowed such a deeply flawed study to even be published. For further information about the errors in the Wax study, and for access to home birth studies, visit understandingbirthbetter.com.

A "scientific study" that amounts to just another offering in US obstetrics' continued propaganda campaign against home birth and autonomous midwifery practice should not fool those who don't base their opinions solely on headlines, titles, and abstracts and instead read scientific articles critically, even when they are presented in prose that sometimes seems to be deliberately obscure. The three studies that I have discussed above serve as illustrations of how far three US medical journals have strayed from ethical scientific conduct, at least in the field of studies about home birth.

The important message to take away from this, after rejecting all the smoke and mirrors that have been floated out to scare the general public and state legislatures about home birth, is that home birth remains an acceptable alternative to hospital birth for low-risk women who have midwives to assist them, and that such care leads to far fewer medical interventions without sacrificing safety.

NOTES
1. Roy Porter, *The Greatest Benefit to Mankind: A Medical History of Humanity* (New York, London: W. W. Norton, 1997).
2. J. H. Aveling, *English Midwives: Their History and Their Prospects* (London: Churchill, 1872).

3. George Engelmann, *Labor Among Primitive Peoples*, 2nd ed. (St. Louis: J. H. Chambers, 1883). Available electronically at http://etext.virginia.edu/toc/modeng/public/EngLabo.html.

4. A. L. Meenan, I. M. Gaskin, P. Hunt, and C. A. Ball, "A New (Old) Maneuver for the Management of Shoulder Dystocia," *The Journal of Family Practice* 32, no. 6 (1991): 625-629; and Joseph P. Bruner, Susan Drummond, Anna L. Meenan, and Ina May Gaskin, "All-Fours Maneuver for Reducing Shoulder Dystocia in Labor," *The Journal of Reproductive Medicine* 43 (1998): 439-443.

5. Plato, *Timaeus*.

6. Aristotle, *De Generatione Animalium* (Oxford, 1912). See especially II.737a.25 and I.724b, 725a, 725b.

7. Quoted in Simone de Beauvoir, *The Second Sex* (New York: Bantam Books, 1965).

8. Simone de Beauvoir, *The Second Sex* (New York: Bantam Books, 1965).

9. Shulamith Firestone, *The Dialectic of Sex: The Case for Feminist Revolution* (New York: Farrar, Straus and Giroux, 1970).

10. Janet Todd, *Mary Wollstonecraft: A Revolutionary Life* (New York: Columbia University Press, 2002).

11. Elizabeth Cady Stanton, *Eighty Years & More: Reminiscences 1815-1897* (New York: Schocken Books, 1971).

12. Hendrik van Deventer, *The Art of Midwifery Improved, Fully and Plainly Laying Down Whatever Instructions Are Requisite to Make a Compleat Midwife . . . made English from the Latin by an eminent physician*, 3rd ed. (Bettersworth, London: 1728).

13. Jane B. Donegan, *Women & Men Midwives: Medicine, Morality, and Misogyny in Early America* (Westport, CT: Greenwood Press, 1978).

14. Richard M. Wertz and Dorothy C. Wertz, *Lying-In: A History of Childbirth in America*, expanded ed. (New Haven, CT: Yale University Press, 1989).

15. Barbara Ehrenreich and Deirdre English, *For Her Own Good: 150 Years of the Experts' Advice to Women* (Garden City, NY: Anchor Press/Doubleday, 1979); and Anne Llewellyn Barstow, *Witchcraze: A New History of the European Witch Hunts* (San Francisco: Pandora/Harper-Collins, 1994).

16. Carolyn C. van Blarcom, "Rat Pie: Among the Black Midwives of the South," *Harper's Magazine*, February 1930, 322-332.

17. Robert D. Retherford, *The Changing Sex Differential in Mortality* (Westport, CT: Greenwood Press, 1975, 57-69); and Judith Walzer Leavitt, *Brought to Bed: Childbearing in America, 1750-1950* (New York: Oxford University Press, 1986), 182-184.

18. Valerie Lee, *Granny Midwives & Black Women Writers: Double Dutched Readings* (New York and London: Routledge, 1996).

19. Death records of town of Gardner, Massachusetts, 1895-1910, quoted in Eugene R. Declercq, "The Trials of Hanna Porn: The Campaign to Abolish Midwifery in Massachusetts," *American Journal of Public Health* 84 (1994): 1022-1028.

20. Harvey Graham, *Eternal Eve* (London: William Heinemann Medical Books, Ltd., 1950), 376.

21. James Blundell, *The Principles and Practice of Obstetricy* (London: Nabu Press, 1834).

22. Egbert Grandin and George Jarman, *Pregnancy, Labor, and the Puerperal State* (Philadelphia: The F. A. Davis Company, 1895).

23. Harold Speert, *Obstetrics and Gynecology in America: A History* (Chicago: American College of Obstetricians and Gynecologists, 1980).

24. Quoted in Judith Walzer Leavitt, *Brought to Bed: Childbearing in America: 1750-1950* (New York: Oxford University Press, 1986), 105.

25. J. Whitridge Williams, "Medical Education and the Midwife Problem in the United States," *Journal of the American Medical Association* 58 (1912): 1-7.

26. Judith Walzer Leavitt, *Brought to Bed: Childbearing in America, 1750-1950* (New York: Oxford University Press, 1986).

27. Wendy Simonds, Barbara Katz-Rothman, and Bari Meltzer Norman, *Laboring On: Birth in Transition in the United States* (New York: Routledge, Taylor & Francis Group, 2007).

28. George Engelmann, *Labor Among Primitive Peoples* (St. Louis: J. H. Chambers & Son, 1883).

29. Frances Kobrin, "The American Midwife Controversy: A Crisis in Professionalization," *Bulletin on the History of Medicine* 40:350-36; Jean Donnison, *Midwives and Medical Men: A History of Inter-Professional Rivalries and Women's Rights* (New York: Schocken, 1977); and George Engelmann, *Labor among Primitive Peoples* (St. Louis: J. H. Chambers & Son, 1883).

30. Alice Stockham, *Tokology: A Book for Every Woman*, revised ed. (Butler & Tanner, Frome and London, 1891).

31. Gladys Denny Schultz, "Cruelty in the Maternity Wards," *Ladies' Home Journal*, May 1958, 151-155.

32. Ibid.

33. Harold Speert, *Obstetrics and Gynecology in America: A History* (Chicago: American College of Obstetricians and Gynecologists, 1980).

34. Judith P. Rooks, *Midwifery and Childbirth in America* (Philadelphia: Temple University Press, 1997).

35. Ibid.

36. Tom Kisken, "Rally Protests Camarillo Hospital's Decision to Ban Midwives," *Ventura County Star*, accessed January 4, 2011, http://www.vcstar.com/news/2010/feb/12/supporters-will-rally-in-oxnard-today-to-protest/.

37. Ed Pilkington, "Home Births Are Driven Underground in New York as Midwives Lose Right to Deliver," *Guardian*, May 15, 2010, 33.

38. L. Saldana, M. E. Rivera-Alsina, J. W. Arias, P. J. Ross, and S. F. Pokorny, "Home Birth: Negative Implications Derived from a Hospital-based Birthing Suite," *Southern Medical Journal* 76, no. 2 (1983): 170-173.

39. M. Lievaart and P. A. de Jong, "Neonatal Morbidity in Deliveries Conducted by Midwives and Gynecologists: A Study of the System of Obstetric Care Prevailing in The Netherlands," *American Journal of Obstetrics and Gynecology* 144, no. 4 (1982): 376-386.

40. P. E. Treffers and D. van Alten, "Condemnation of Obstetric Care in The Netherlands?" *American Journal of Obstetrics and Gynecology* 146, no. 7 (1983): 871-874.

41. Lievaart and de Jong, "Neonatal Morbidity," 376.

42. E. Declercq, Marian F. MacDorman, Fay Menacker, and Naomi Stotland, "Characteristics of Planned and Unplanned Home Births in 19 States," *Obstetrics and Gynecology* 116, no. 1 (2010): 93-99.

43. J. W. Pang, J. D. Heffelfinger, G. J. Huang, T. J. Benedetti, and N. S. Weiss, "Outcomes of Planned Home Births in Washington State: 1989-1996," *Obstetrics and Gynecology* 100, no. 2 (2002): 253-259.

44. J. R. Wax, F. L. Lucas, M. Lamont, M. G. Pinette, A. Cartin, and J. Blackstone, "Maternal and Newborn Outcomes in Planned Home Birth vs Planned Hospital Births: A Meta-analysis," *American Journal of Obstetrics and Gynecology* 203, no. 3 (2010): 243.e1–e8.

45. American Congress of Obstetricians and Gynecologists, ACOG Statement of Policy: Home Births in the United States. Available at http://www.acog.org/publications/policy_statements/sop705.cfm, (accessed on January 27, 2009).

46. *The Lancet*, "Home Birth-Proceed with Caution, 376, no. 9738 (July 2010): 303, doi:10.1016/S0140-6736(10)61165-8.

47. Personal communication: Saraswathi Vedam, etc.

48. A. de Jonge, B. Y. van der Goes, A. C. J. Ravelli, M. P. Amelink-Verburg, B. W. Mol, J. G. Nijhuis, J. Bennebroeck Gravenhorst, and S. E. Buitendijk, "Perinatal Mortality and Morbidity in a Nationwide Cohort of 529,688 Low-risk Planned Home and Hospital Births," *British Journal of Obstetrics and Gynaecology* 116, no. 9 (2009): 1177–1184.

49. T. Dowswell, J. G. Thornton, J. Hewison, R. J. Lilford, J. Raisler, A. Macfarlane, G. Young, M. Newburn, R. Dodds, and R. S. Settatree, "Should There Be a Trial of Home versus Hospital Delivery in the United Kingdom?" *British Medical Journal* 321, no. 7033 (1996): 753–757.

50. K. Johnson and B. A. Daviss, "Outcomes of Planned Home Births with Certified Professional Midwives: Large Prospective Study in North America," *British Medical Journal* 330, no. 7505 (2005): 1416–1419.

51. H. C. Woodcock, A. W. Read, C. Bower, F. J. Stanley, and D. J. Moore, "A Matched Cohort Study of Planned Home and Hospital Births in Western Australia 1981-1987," *Midwifery* 10 (1994): 125–135.

52. H. E. Lindgren, I. J. Radestad, K. Christensson, and I. M. Hildengsson, "Outcomes of Planned Home Births Compared to Hospital Births in Sweden Between 1992 and 2004: A Population-based Register Study," *Acta Obstetricia et Gynecologica Scandinavia* 87, no. 7 (2008): 751–759.

53. J. M. L. Shearer, Five Year Prospective Survey of Risk of Booking for a Home Birth in Essex," *British Medical Journal* 219 (1985): 1478–1480.

54. Richard Horton, "Offline: Urgency and Concern about Home Births," *The Lancet* 376, no. 9755 (November 27, 2010): 1812.

Chloe at The Farm

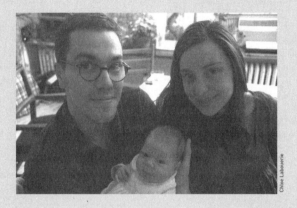

Chloe Labouerie

I woke-up suddenly early one morning with a very sharp and brief contraction. Having never felt one before, it startled me so much that I literally jumped out of bed! But it only lasted a few seconds, and I quickly forgot about it. The rest of the morning went as usual: I went for an hour-long walk with Charles, my husband, and then practiced yoga.

At 1:00 PM we went to the clinic for my weekly check-up with Carol. She said that my cervix was almost completely thinned out and that I was dilated to 3 cm—the baby would certainly come in the next couple of days! Charles and I sat with Carol for a few minutes and asked her all sorts of questions (When will the baby come? What do people do with the placenta?). She had a slight grin on her face, as though she knew something was going to happen but didn't want to give us false hopes! When we left I was very uncomfortable: I had a lot of cramping but thought nothing of it.

We got into the car to head home, but we didn't get very far before I had to get out and walk. It was just impossible for me to sit down because my back ached so much with each bump of the road.

As I stepped out of the car, a female dog appeared out of nowhere and started following me, a few steps behind, until I reached the cottage where we were staying. She had such a gentle attitude. Looking back, I think she knew that something was about to happen . . .

My mother, who was staying with us in the cottage, and had driven with us from New York, had prepared lunch. I was very hungry. I kept getting up from the table every few minutes to go outside where I could walk around and stretch my body, and then I would go back inside, sit down, and try to resume eating. The sensation wouldn't let me eat in peace! It was not really painful per say, just uncomfortable, and I couldn't stop the urge to move around. I kept sitting down again and trying to finish my lunch because I thought it would pass. I absolutely did not think for one second that I was going into labor.

My mother and Charles wanted to call Carol, but I didn't think it was happening and did not want to give false alarm. After maybe half an hour of this going back and forth, I started to feel real contractions. I went to the bedroom and focused on deep breathing. I tried lying down because I was a bit tired, but it definitely felt better to stand up or squat.

Eventually, Charles came into the room, sat next to me, and started timing me. The contractions were all about three minutes apart and lasted for forty-five seconds. They were getting progressively stronger. Really strong.

There is no way I will be able to stand this for twenty hours, I thought.

I got scared, and Charles ran out to fetch Carol.

Maybe twenty minutes passed, which seemed like eternity because the contractions were so strong. *Where is Carol? Why is this going so fast? How can I go on like this?*

I felt awful. I started gagging when Charles came back and he ran to get a bucket. I threw-up and immediately felt better. My stomach wasn't weighing on the baby anymore, so I felt lighter.

Carol arrived and set up some things in the room. Then, she pulled up a chair and sat. Charles and my mother took chairs as well and watched me. It was strange because I felt like a circus animal or a science experiment with three people just watching me. It wasn't a very pleasant feeling at that particular moment, so I tried to shut them out in order to focus on breathing deeply.

Inhale and open—exhale and open more. Don't resist. Don't frown.

I kept saying those words over and over again in my mind like a mantra. The contractions were quite strong and close together. I was getting used to the feeling, and felt like I was "managing" them. I would squat each time, which I found helped a lot.

Suddenly, the feeling shifted. I felt a very small urge to push during the contractions, while I was squatting. I was not sure how to manage it all, and started to feel overwhelmed . . . I needed to be more focused to keep up!

I wanted to be alone with Carol, so I could look deep into her face and let her eyes guide me. I asked Charles and my mother to leave the room, which they did, reluctantly, but without any argument.

Once alone with Carol I could not speak much, but I told her that things were "changing." When she checked me I was eight centimeters dilated—what a relief! It felt great to know that I had made so much progress.

She asked if I wanted to try the birthing chair and I immediately agreed. I sat on the chair and ripped off my dress. I was completely drenched in sweat by that time. I was pushing a little during each contraction and suddenly something came flying out like a balloon.

Wow that was easy, and it did not even hurt?

But it was only my water breaking! Carol reassured me that this was all fine. She was so reassuring every step of the way. I think if you trust in birth the way she does, it just emanates from you and gives women confidence.

With each new contraction, when I pushed, I could feel the baby's weight shifting down. My back ached a lot, so Carol gently massaged it with some oil. It really helped. But the contractions were short and I did not have time to push hard enough. Each time I released the pressure, the baby would go back up. Carol reassured me that this was normal, and told me not to be discouraged.

I tried getting on the floor on my hands and knees. The first time I let out a sound that really startled me. It was a very deep and very loud roar like an animal. *Where did that come from?* The famous primal scream!

This went on for maybe ten contractions. No progress. And then a strange thing happened: the contractions stopped.

COMPLETELY.

I felt no pain at all, but was so very tired. And scared. Scared that I would have no energy left and that I would end up in the hospital with a C-section because I was too weak to push anymore. *How could they just stop? This is not supposed to happen! I could maybe take a nap and we could start again later?*

I wanted to sleep so badly! I told Carol that the contractions stopped, but she did not seem too concerned. However, she must have sensed that I was distressed because she gave me homeopathy to restart labor.

To my surprise, the contractions started again but they were not very strong and I was getting tired and desperate. Carol suggested I try getting on the bed. I did and it felt great to be able to lean back into the pillows to rest in between the rushes. Still, I was not making any progress, and I went from being scared and tired to being angry. I decided I would push with every bit of strength I had left and get it over with! I grabbed my knees and pushed as much as I could, and the baby started crowning. But then the contractions stopped and she went back in again. But the next time, I pushed just a little bit in between, just to keep her where she was and not lose all the work I had done. It took about another three sets of contractions before I was able to push hard enough to get the head halfway through.

At that point Carol, placed a mirror under me so I could see the baby's head, which was very encouraging. Then she warned me that it would burn and probably be painful, but that all the stinging did not necessarily mean that there was a tear. She said that I shouldn't worry about that. I just needed to push right through that sensation.

She was right. I felt a sharp sting. I was pushing as hard as I possibly could. I don't remember how long that lasted—just pushing with each contraction, with my eyes shut tight. I was very tired and in another space I think. Just drifting away.

I was startled when Carol suddenly gave me the order: "REACH DOWN AND HELP PULL HER OUT, CHLOE!" *What? How? But I'm too weak . . .*

I snapped out of my strange journey and somehow I leaned forward and grabbed my baby and pulled her out. Carol helped to pull her onto my chest. I asked her to please call Charles and my mother and they came rushing over, along with another midwife named Sharon who was waiting with them on the porch.

We stayed like this for a very long time. It was wonderful. She cried very softly and moved her adorable little arms.

A few minutes later the placenta came out very easily, and Carol checked me: I had no tear. Sharon helped me place the baby at my breast and she immediately latched on. What a relief! I had been quite nervous about it. I thought I might have trouble breastfeeding.

Annabelle was born at 7:00 PM. I had labored for only five hours. It took a little over a half an hour to push her out. It was the perfect birth I was looking for.

—Chloe Labouerie

CHAPTER 5

Technology and Empowerment

Things are in the saddle and ride mankind.
—Ralph Waldo Emerson

It is easy for people to imagine that medical technologies and new drugs have been created and improved in maternity care at the same pace as they have been in other areas of life—to imagine that we now have drugs that can somehow enable babies to be born without putting their mothers through transformative changes. The truth is that the new developments in the area of obstetrics and maternity care that have appeared over the last generation are primarily those within the realm of fertility medicine, out-of-body conception, and the ability to peek inside the uterus. I'm referring to in vitro fertilization, the harvesting of eggs, blastocyst implantation, drugs to stimulate ovulation, implanting pregnancies in postmenopausal women, and the technology of ultrasound. Such innovations have nothing to do with getting babies out of their mothers in safer, less challenging ways than nature provides for. Implanted babies-to-be, once they've sufficiently matured inside a woman's body, must still be born. This means that the ancient processes are still relevant—unless they are entirely bypassed by surgery (as they too often are).

Uteri and vaginas are not like ill-functioning hearts, which, when they become sick, can have their clogged valves or arteries surgically reopened, at least temporarily, or eyes whose vision can sometimes be greatly improved by cataract or laser surgery. There's no tinkering with the uterus in this way. We should make every effort possible not to damage it. We need to recognize that technology is humbled in some very important ways by pregnancy and birth. Many of our current problems in US maternity care stem from the fact that we leave no room for recognizing when nature is smarter than we are.

HOW TECHNOLOGY CHANGES KNOWLEDGE AND PRACTICE IN BIRTH

When I began working as a midwife in the early seventies, the usual way of diagnosing pregnancy involved placing the hands on the woman's abdomen and feeling the size of the uterus. We called this "palpation," and we did (and still do) it not only to diagnose pregnancy, but also throughout pregnancy to determine a baby's position, the amount of amniotic fluid, how the woman is carrying the baby, and the baby's weight. Midwives have been performing this kind of assessment for as long as there have been humans, but the skill acquired its medical name, "Leopold's Maneuvers," when a Dr. Leopold (in the 1880s) described four distinct actions that make up this skill. For hundreds of years, every doctor, every obstetric nurse, and every midwife was supposed to know Leopold's Maneuvers.

Fast forward to 2002. I was scanning an obstetrical journal when an article title caught my eye. "Predicting Fetal Weight: Are Leopold's Maneuvers Still Worth Teaching to Medical Students and House Staff?" The author concluded that yes, palpation was still a worthwhile skill to teach medical students, because his study showed that experienced physicians could make more accurate predictions of babies' weights using palpation than could medical students.[1]

I was mildly relieved that this study showed the value of retaining a time-honored and essential manual skill but surprised to learn that some teaching hospitals had already stopped teaching it because its usefulness had been challenged by the advent of modern ultrasonographic techniques for predicting fetal weight. This could be compared to pilots being taught to rely only on electronic systems for flying, taking off, and landing, rather than being taught manual skills as well (which can be useful if the electronics malfunction). Couldn't they have thought about it a little longer before deciding to stop the teaching of an ancient skill? The idea that it is good to forget about teaching practical skills because of new technology has always rubbed me the wrong way. People who care for pregnant and laboring women—whether they are midwives, nurses, or physicians—should not have ignorant hands. I suspected that sooner or later someone would suffer for the lack of knowledge that would result from a total reliance on ultrasonography during pregnancy.

An especially egregious example of what I'm talking about happened in November 2008 in Cape Fear, North Carolina. A news report from a local television station caught my attention. It seems that a woman was subjected to a C-section during which the obstetrician, who cut into her abdomen, discovered that she wasn't even pregnant. According to that obstetrician, "several doctors had examined and attempted to induce labor on the patient for several days before the C-section incident."[2] Not one of them seems to have manually checked the accuracy of the diagnosis of pregnancy; the intern who looked at the woman's ultrasound and found no heart beat had assumed that "the baby" had died, failing to take into account that sometimes there is no baby inside a woman who thinks she is pregnant and has some superficial signs of pregnancy.

Any physician practicing obstetrics should know of pseudocyesis (false pregnancy), but so many doctors today rely solely on imaging technologies that they forget to keep their manual techniques and their thinking skills as sharp as they need to be (or they even forget to apply their hands to a woman's abdomen). One obstetrician in an electronic discussion of this bizarre group mistake guessed that the intern who "diagnosed" the pregnancy had probably mistaken retained fecal material for a baby. I found that comment amusing, since I've never once felt an accumulation of poop in the shape of a baby. However, I *have* diagnosed two false pregnancies without ultrasound, one of them during my first few months of caring for pregnant women. Hands are still useful— even in the era of ultrasound. A simple, hand-on-the-belly palpation for uterine size (a nonpregnant uterus usually can't even be felt) is all that would be necessary. My recommendation is that all medical schools get back to teaching Leopold's Maneuvers and other manual skills (including the art of the painless vaginal exam) that are a necessary part of the skill set that belongs to maternity care. It's bizarre and sad that doctors have become so disinterested in the old ways of treating pregnant women that students are no longer taught the skills of palpation, how to perform a vaginal exam without causing pain, or external turning of a breech baby to a headfirst position.

The same deficiencies in education and training also apply to many nurses who plan to work in maternity wards. An increasing number of them graduate from nursing schools without ever having been exposed to the skills (that go beyond machine-tending) that are relevant to looking after laboring women—the same skills that most people imagine that these students would be required to master during their training. Nurses often tell me that they come out of nursing school better prepared to care for geriatric patients than laboring women, because in many teaching hospitals there are far more elderly patients than there are women who manage to give birth vaginally (while being observed by a class of nurses). I have lost count of how many newly graduated nurses have told me in recent months that they had never been in a room with a laboring woman before they were hired as a hospital maternity nurse. I still feel shocked at how widespread the educational philosophy of see one, do one, teach one is in medicine and nursing. Would we throw student pilots into situations like this

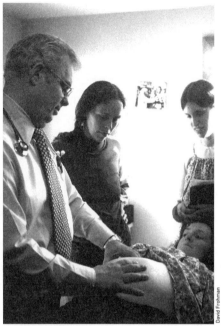

Dr. John D. Williams, Jr. showing me his method for detecting a breech.

and expect them to perform well? Obviously not, because each student pilot's teacher actually has to be up in the air with the student. And, just like the student pilot, in the case of the student nurse or doctor lives are at stake. Why are we not more careful in how we prepare medical professionals for providing maternity care? Better apprenticeships would seem to be in order. We should make this a national priority.

Midwifery students in countries with superior maternity services (as measured by maternal and infant outcomes) are taught the skills of abdominal palpation, pelvic and cervical examination, assessment of intensity of labor, and distinguishing between ordinary labor pain and the labor pain that signals a complication, and they must demonstrate their competence if they are to receive the certification or registration that allows them to be employed in the hospitals of their respective countries.

In the US, we force obstetric nurses to learn on the job, without being routinely taught about nonpharmacologic pain relief, and often without a mentor present in the room. Instead of providing continuous care for one woman, the beginning nurse will typically be expected to care for at least three or four laboring women simultaneously. Since the 1990s, many US hospitals have required their maternity nurses to care for more laboring women than was previously considered safe or possible. Many nurses get bladder infections because of the difficulty in finding the time to take a bathroom break. It's now a common complaint that the nurse pays more attention to the monitor than to the laboring woman. No wonder so many women are hiring doulas, who do have the skills that maternity nurses used to be taught for helping women to labor as comfortably and effectively as possible without resorting to numbing medication. Women who cannot afford to hire a doula are often placed in situations in which it is nearly impossible for labor to progress in a way that isn't traumatizing.

The Cape Fear incident (a national embarrassment, to say the least) is just one example of how the overenthusiastic use of a technology can cause maternity caregivers to become ignorant of other ways of knowing. However, there *are* other ways.

My friend, the late Margaret Charles Smith, author of *Listen to Me Good: The Life Story of an Alabama Midwife*, told me that during her years of work as an Alabama "registered" midwife, the rules established by the health department specified that midwives were not allowed to have fetoscopes for listening to babies' heart rates. That didn't matter to her, though, because she could put her hands on a woman's belly, locate, and feel the baby's pulse. I have known US obstetricians who were surprised to know that the standard "acoustic" tool for listening to babies' heart rates in most European countries is a Pinard Horn fetoscope, a small metal or wooden cone with a flattened top on the ear end. Unthinking contempt for older, simpler forms of technology is as silly as abandoning past wisdom about what hands can do.

Sometimes, wise women, realizing that even some experienced doctors would benefit from having their minds rearranged, find ways to teach them what they should have been taught during medical school. A childbirth educator friend of mine told me about Nicole, who managed to teach her obstetrician a kind of humility that he hadn't yet learned. She had gone to him for her first two births, but had not been satisfied with how they had gone. At the same time, she liked and respected the man as a person.

"I'm going to ask you to attend this last birth," she told him, "but *only if you do not touch me while it is happening.*" Without argument, he agreed to her condition and kept to her terms. Mind you, this was a hospital birth, but instead of doing vaginal examinations every now and then and performing an episiotomy, he merely held his hands so that the baby could fall into them. This man, who had seen so many births already and was considered within the dominant birth culture as an authority on birth, was moved to tears by seeing a woman give birth in ecstasy, with her full power evident. This was a Saul of Tarsus moment for him; never before had he witnessed an ecstatic birth, nor had an inkling that birth could be anything but an ordeal for a woman.

WHEN THERE IS LITTLE OR NO VAGINAL BIRTH

Most people don't consider that the way in which women give birth in hospitals affects what physicians, midwives, and nurses know about birth and its possibilities. Those whose training and work occurs exclusively in hospitals, with high rates of medical intervention, may view alternative methods of care as harmful. As just described, due to the routine use of high-tech devices and diagnostic equipment, obstetrical skills that were once considered vital are often no longer taught in the US.

It seems that we are rapidly approaching the situation that Brazil has had for many years, with its extremely high rates of C-sections in private hospitals. I once met a Brazilian obstetrician who was thought by his colleagues to be a radical because he had begun attending home births. He told me that there was a woman who had planned to have her first baby at home with him, but that her baby was lying crosswise in her uterus. He asked me if I would be willing to try to turn this baby so the woman could avoid a C-section. I agreed, and the woman, accompanied by her husband, lay down. The doctor began putting his video camera on a tripod so he would have a record of the procedure. Meanwhile, there I was, looking awkwardly at the woman, since she didn't speak English, and I didn't speak Portuguese. When words don't work, there's always touch, so my hand reached out to touch her belly to see where the head was, and I accidentally pushed the baby's head hard enough to turn the baby. "You didn't wait for me to turn on the camera!" the obstetrician protested. "I didn't know it was going to be that easy," I told him. What fascinated me was what happens to the mind of the professional when the psychology of fear sets in. Common sense goes. The professional caregiver literally gets "out of touch."

I find it sad that obstetrics has been so dumbed down in the US that few doctors are taught anymore how to deal with a vaginal breech birth. They especially fear the case in which the baby's feet present before its head. The very prospect frightens many because they have never witnessed a breech birth. This fact really came home to me in the early eighties when I was invited to show videos and speak to ob-gyn residents at a medical school in North Carolina. Just before introducing me, the department chairman who had invited me to speak whispered, "Do you realize that you and I are the only people in this room who have ever witnessed a breech birth?" What astounded me was the speed of the change in the very content of the obstetrics curriculum. When I learned that the reason for such a change was insurance companies that began threatening teaching hospitals during the seventies and eighties that they would deny them malpractice coverage if they provided opportunities for residents to witness a breech birth attended by an experienced practitioner, I had to wonder if doctors of the future would ever regain such skills. These skills, by the way, could easily be taught using pelvic models and dolls in the way that breech skills are still taught in medical schools in other parts of the world.

Why should insurance companies continue to get away with limiting the skills that a health profession had always previously required of its members if they were to be considered fully trained? I know of at least two maternal deaths that happened in recent years in the US because of fear and ignorance surrounding vaginal breech birth. In both cases, the physician chose a C-section because of the breech presentation. In one case, the mother died from hemorrhage during the emergency C-section performed for her second twin, whose feet presented, along with the umbilical cord, after her first baby had been vaginally born. This is the one case of umbilical cord prolapse that is *not* dangerous, because it doesn't pinch the cord between the baby's body and that of the mother, and a footling breech born with "the door already open" should be easily accomplished if the doctor or midwife is not petrified with fear. In effect, a mother of eight died because of ignorance that was imposed on her doctor by the insurance industry. I find this intolerable.

The second maternal death was that of a family practice physician, whose second C-section (her first C-section had been scheduled only because of a breech presentation) was complicated by an accidental nick of her bowel, which went untreated too long and caused her to die from septic shock.

I related my concerns about the rising rates of C-section and induction at a clinical conference for obstetricians at Sarasota Memorial Hospital in 2009. Florida, by the way, is one of the few US states that has made strong efforts to conduct maternal mortality reviews in recent years. At the conclusion of my talk, which included full information about my unusual path to midwifery, how I was able to learn valuable techniques from indigenous people, why I promote sphincter law as a key to understanding the physiology of birth, and a look at some of the stories that have come to me because of the Safe Motherhood Quilt Project, which I will discuss later, I invited questions from my audience of obstetricians. A distinguished-looking man from the front row announced in a loud voice that the C-section rate in the Miami area had just risen above 50 percent, and turning around to face his colleagues, he declared, "and I think that everyone in this room knows that this is going to cause more maternal deaths." After the conclusion of the conference, an obstetrician told me that he thought I could do more for women by going out and speaking to groups of physicians than I could if I devoted my time primarily to attending births. My answer was that I love speaking to obstetricians and family physicians who do obstetrics, and continue to welcome invitations to do so.

THE ELECTRONIC MONITORING CRAZE

The equipment used for electronic fetal monitoring (EFM) during labor was enthusiastically bought by every hospital in the country soon after its development in the sixties, with the belief that early detection of a change in the baby's heart rate would lower the death rate for newborns. What happened instead was that C-section rates rose because of physicians' problems in interpreting what the new equipment revealed. Many babies, erroneously thought to be in trouble during labor, were delivered by C-section, and then found to be perfectly all right. What physicians hadn't counted on was the lowered fetal heart rates during uterine contractions that could be picked up for the first time with the continuous monitor, and that were absolutely normal. An additional problem for laboring women was that the monitors required them to lie flat on their backs for best reception. Before electronic monitoring became routine, it was common for laboring women in small hospitals (in which twilight sleep wasn't the norm) to walk around as much as they liked during the first part of labor. This movement not only made labor less painful and boring, it helped babies move into the positions more favorable for being born.

EFM, then, had the unintended effect of making labor far more painful than it had been, so the epidural began to be used routinely in most hospitals. The epidural, especially when given early in labor, tends to increase the length of labor. For this reason, it became common to augment the strength and pace of contractions with intravenous synthetic oxytocin (such as Pitocin). The synthetic oxytocin causes severe contractions that can sometimes reduce blood flow to the baby for longer than natural contractions would. The problem introduced by this practice produced, once again, an increase in the number of cases of fetal distress leading to a C-section.

The scientific evidence is clear that intermittent listening with a fetoscope is just as reliable as EFM.[3] The difference is that one requires more human contact than the other, so in a profit-oriented system such as that in the US, we know which is more likely. Electronic fetal monitors don't need health insurance or salaries, while midwives and nurses do.

If the evidence is strong that electronic monitoring doesn't reduce the death rate of babies but does increase the C-section rate, you may wonder why it continues to be used. The answer is pretty silly, because it has to do with appearances. The long strips of paper records that are produced by electronic fetal monitors after each woman's labor make it possible for hospitals or clinicians to defend themselves in court. They create the appearance that someone is constantly aware of the baby's well-being throughout labor. Many hospitals take advantage of this appearance by reducing the amount of time the midwife or maternity nurse is actually able to spend with each laboring mother by requiring them to care for more women simultaneously than was previously thought safe. Good maternity care actually requires attentive, well-trained, calm, and compassionate humans who know a lot about the physiology of labor. No amount of new electronic equipment can ever fill this need. Good maternity care also requires continuous one-on-one attention. Laboring women—especially those having their first vaginal birth—should not have to share their midwife or nurse with several other women.

THE POWER TO PEEK

Those technologies that provide glimpses inside the uterus are especially beguiling. When X-rays were first introduced into the medical arsenal during the early twentieth century, they were used for locating shrapnel or bullets in gunshot wounds or for looking at fractures before setting broken bones. Very quickly, well-meaning doctors and dentists began using them for all sorts of other conditions, including tonsillitis, ringworm, respiratory problems, and acne. Even owners of shoe stores were quick to purchase the new technology. I can remember going shopping with my mother in 1950, where the store owner was proudly showing off his new X-ray machine, the newest "scientific" tool for making sure that shoes fit. My mother wisely kept my siblings and me from sticking our feet into the machine, since she couldn't understand how seeing the bones in one's feet was better than just trying the shoes on. She used to tell me that people from Missouri (meaning herself) are like that. I remember meeting a woman a few years later who suffered from severe radiation burns that she had gotten from X-ray treatments for her fingernail fungus. She was sorry that she had trusted her doctor's assurances that he gave only safe treatments.

Obstetricians began using X-rays for a variety of imagined benefits: to stimulate ovulation, diagnose pregnancy, estimate fetal maturity, rule out skeletal abnormalities in babies, examine the placenta, and measure babies' heads and mothers' pelvises. I say "imagined," because X-rays don't stimulate ovaries to ovulate, are useless for estimating fetal maturity, and don't reveal any useful information about the condition of the placenta in most cases. There are far less harmful ways of diagnosing pregnancy. And as for having any predictive value about the size of the baby relative to the mother's pelvic size—complete nonsense.

The big problem with X-ray images—the one that stopped their carefree experimental use—was the cancer they caused. Even then, though, there was a lag before patterns were changed. Despite the mounting evidence of the dangers of ionizing radiation after the nuclear bombs were dropped on Hiroshima and Nagasaki in 1945, the known high incidence of infertility among X-ray technicians, and the meticulous research on 16 million English and Welsh children published in 1958 by Dr. Alice Stewart and her colleagues that showed a doubling of childhood cancers from prenatal exposure to radiation at levels of one-fiftieth to one-hundredth of those assumed as "safe" by the medical establishment,[4] a major US obstetrical textbook published in 1965 still dismissed the "fear and hysteria of radiation damage" as insignificant. Its author based his opinion on the wishful thought that the babies' gonads would be protected against radiation "by the uterus, amniotic fluid and the abdominal wall of the mother."[5] Of course, the mother's body offered no such protection against radiation.

By the late seventies, ultrasound machines, which first became available in 1963, had replaced X-ray technology as a routine part of obstetric care. Most obstetricians were happy to proceed on the assumption that the new technology would have no harmful effects on the developing embryo or fetus, simply because ultrasound aims high-frequency sound waves, not ionizing radiation, at the tissues, and not because of any evidence showing that the routine use of ultrasound could lower the death rate of babies. Some scientists in the field of radiology and imagery did express their concerns about the lack of an evidence-based approach in the acceptance of this new technology. H. D. Meier, a UK radiologist, commented in 1987:

> The casual observer might be forgiven for wondering why the medical profession is now involved in the wholesale examination of pregnant patients with machines emanating vastly different powers of energy which is not proven to be harmless to obtain information which is not proven to be of any clinical value by operators who are not certified as competent to perform the operation.[6]

None of these factors has changed since that comment was made. In fact, in the US, where Food and Drug Administration (FDA) regulations have been loosened to allow unborn babies to be exposed to intensities eight times higher than previously allowed, caution has been thrown to the wind, and anyone in the US willing to fork over the cash can buy an ultrasound machine. Actor Tom Cruise, who bought one when his wife became pregnant so they could have a look at their developing baby whenever they wanted throughout the pregnancy, was not the only untrained person to believe unlimited exposure to ultrasound harmless.

While we still have no way to know about any long-term effects of the routine and casual use of ultrasound, we do know that exposure does heat mammalian tissue (including the developing organs of embryos), and that its vibrations pop little bubbles of gas in living tissue. It would seem wise that we try to limit the use of ultrasound when our knowledge of its long-term impact is so incomplete. Large studies carried out in Denmark have shown an increased tendency toward left-handedness in babies exposed to ultrasound in utero. Additionally, there are a number of studies that have suggested that the heating and collapsing of gas bubbles in developing mammalian tissue may not be harmless. One study published in the early nineties showed cell abnormalities caused by exposure to ultrasound that were seen to persist for several generations.[7] Here in the US, there is little incentive to do such research, since research can be expensive and no one would profit more than they already do from it.

I mentioned above how seductive X-ray technology was. Ultrasound is even more so, because of the chance it gives to pregnant women to learn the baby's gender. Do I ever advocate its use? Yes. There are instances when an ultrasound is medically called for, such as to determine if twins in utero are protected from entanglement of their respective umbilical cords by a layer of membrane between them. It can also be helpful in determining the location of the placenta in a woman who had a previous uterine surgery, information that could be relevant to her choice of how to give birth in the future. However, I adhere to the precautionary principle, under which a new drug or treatment is considered unsafe until it's proven safe, so I continue to think it's a good idea to try to limit the number of ultrasounds in any given pregnancy.

INDUCTION

There are legitimate reasons for the induction of labor, but rates of induction greater than 10 percent of all births are excessive. Cancer, hypertension, diabetes, kidney disease, significant intrauterine growth retardation in a baby, a significant decrease in amniotic fluid (diagnosed manually), or an intrauterine fetal death followed by a long wait for labor to begin (we're talking three weeks or so, not days) are all legitimate reasons for induction. However, inductions should not be done for nonmedical reasons, because they can be dangerous to both mothers and babies. The dangers include maternal and fetal death due to amniotic fluid embolism or ruptured uterus. Induced labors are much more painful than labors that begin spontaneously, and they lead more often to C-sections as well.

Babies often suffer from induced labors, from distress caused by the unnaturally hard contractions and from prematurity (caused by mistaken estimation of the baby's actual gestational age). It is a sad fact that inductions are not always performed because it is thought best for the mother or baby, but because it allows births to be scheduled for those hours when it is more convenient for medical staff—the daylight hours on Monday through Friday.[8]

A sordid history is exposed when you consider the widespread use in the 1990s of the popular drug Cytotec (generic name: misoprostol). The manufacturer warned from the beginning that it should not be used on pregnant women. Yet, obstetricians used it regularly to induce labor, ultimately killing more than one hundred mothers in the US, according to the Food and Drug Administration, and even more babies.[9] Today, physicians around the country continue to use this dangerous drug to induce labor, without ever telling the women that the drug is not FDA-approved for this purpose. Cytotec might be useful in obstetrics to stop post-birth hemorrhage, for which purpose it has been proven effective and has shown no risk for women, but its continued use to induce labor is unacceptable.

I watch the television birth stories on satellite television enough to know that many women are no longer being informed about the risks of having their labors induced when they are still only thirty-seven or thirty-eight weeks pregnant. Babies born before thirty-nine weeks often have immature lungs and respiratory problems, and are more susceptible to infection. Such early inductions often end up as C-sections, since neither the baby nor the mother's body is truly ready for birth.

EPIDURALS

Epidurals, as good as they are compared with earlier forms of pain-numbing medications (and I would certainly want one if I had to undergo abdominal surgery), aren't perfect for women in labor. In about 10 percent of cases, they don't provide good pain relief.[10] In about 5 percent of cases, the epidural catheter has to be reinserted.[11] Epidurals inhibit beta-endorphin and oxytocin release, and this means that they interfere with the mother's ability to move into the ecstatic state of consciousness that is a part of normal labor—the "mommy brain," as some have called it. These hormones, which peak at birth in both mother and baby, also help the mother and baby to fall in love with each other in the first moments after birth.

Epidurals are popular among US women because they numb labor pain without causing amnesia or loss of consciousness. Hospitals favor them because when epidurals are used, the mothers are monitored with electronic fetal monitoring, meaning that one nurse or midwife watches the monitors of several women simultaneously. Instead of each woman having a midwife or nurse with her to encourage and support her throughout labor, the maternity ward functions with lower staffing levels, saving the hospital the cost of salaries and benefits for more nurses or midwives. The savings, of course, are not passed to laboring mothers, who are left with the beeping machines instead of human companionship.

Epidurals do have unintended side effects:

- They can make it harder for the mother to push her baby out, since she can no longer feel what is happening in the part of her body that matters most.
- They significantly increase the likelihood of forceps or vacuum extractors being used, thereby increasing the risk of vaginal or perineal trauma that may lead to sexual problems or later incontinence.
- They often significantly increase the length of labor.[12]
- Most women who have epidurals are unable to walk, so their labors are no longer helped by gravity. (Try to imagine how easy it would be to poop while lying down. It's a similar problem.)
- Epidurals make it difficult for the baby who is not already poised to move out of the uterus at the most favorable angle to correct

its position, since they cause most women to have to lie completely still.

- In about one women in every five, the epidural causes a fever, which cannot be readily distinguished from that caused by intrauterine infection. This means a painful septic workup for the baby, involving several needle jabs and sometimes a spinal tap, and nearly always some degree of separation from the mother.
- Epidurals almost always cause a dramatic drop in blood pressure (hypotension), so women who will be given an epidural are first loaded with IV fluids to lessen the fetal distress involved with hypotension.
- Women for whom the epidural gives strong pain relief may be injured by improper positioning by inattentive caregivers (usually, this involves the woman's legs being sharply flexed at the hips while she lies on her back and pushes), since injury is not felt by the woman when it is taking place.
- Rarely, an epidural can result in a maternal death or permanent paralysis. Out of 350 cases of maternal death in the US that I was able to gather for the database of the Safe Motherhood Quilt Project, discussed below, I have found at least four that were caused by epidural analgesia or anesthesia.[13]

Despite their potential drawbacks, epidurals can sometimes be a good idea for women in labor. Sometimes labor is well advanced, but the mother is exhausted from having labored for many hours and needs a rest in order to regain the necessary strength to become fully dilated and push her baby out. In cases like this, an epidural can sometimes be the factor that makes a vaginal birth possible, by giving the mother a break from the pain of labor that allows for the last bit of cervical dilation to take place.

THE COST OF TOO MUCH SURGERY

When people get in the habit of living in a way that is quite alienated from nature, birth also can be more perilous for mothers and babies than it needs to be. I'm writing this book at a time in human history when women in the urban areas of an increasing number of countries are being pushed into surgical births as the preferred way for babies to come into the world. The US C-section rate in 1970 was 5.5 percent of all births; only ten years later, it had quadrupled, with no perceptible benefit for mothers or babies. In 2008, the rate was 32.3 percent.

It is possible to look at other areas of health care in which unnecessary surgery became fashionable for a while before a more rational approach won out. The frequent use of lobotomy for certain mental disorders and the "prophylactic" tonsillectomy that was popular during the 1940s and 1950s are examples of surgeries that are no longer as fashionable as they once were. British historian G. J. Barker-Benfield's important book *The Horrors of the Half-Known Life*, first published in 1974, examined the "ferocious competitiveness with other men" that led many nineteenth-century US doctors to perform unnecessary surgery on women—what anyone today would consider outright mutilation if it had been carried out in another country. A woman who was thought to have masturbated or possibly had a jealous husband was considered to have a dangerous mental disorder, and the cure was clitoridectomy (surgical removal of the clitoris), a practice that began in the 1860s in certain areas of the US and ended only in the early twentieth century. The removal of perfectly healthy ovaries and uteri (hysterectomies) was even more common.[14] Barker-Benfield was shocked at the aggressive surgical practices that were carried out on US women (which would not have been considered acceptable in England and on the European continent), and quoted many US doctors who proudly wrote about their surgical experiments on women. I'm glad to say that a new edition of his book was finally published in 2000.

An unpleasant truth about maternal mortality finally came to the attention of the US media in 2010. California reported a near tripling in its maternal death rate between 1996 and 2006, attributing part of the sudden rise to an excess of cesarean sections.[15] After declining for decades, the maternal mortality rate in New York began to go up in the late 1990s, approximately doubling the previous rates. The same trend occurred in Florida as well. Are increases in C-sections and maternal death rates related to each other? According to what obstetrician Arthur Fougner, the commissioner of government affairs for New York's Medical Society, told investigative reporter Mary Beth Pfeiffer, the answer is yes. "The maternal death rate is rising, in part, because of the increased number of surgical deliveries," he said.[16]

US women today face at least double the chance of dying from pregnancy or birth-related causes than their mothers did. The British journal *The Lancet* published an article that detailed how nearly all of 181 countries studied had lowered their rates of maternal death. However, the article went on to say that in four countries— the US, Canada, Norway, and Afghanistan—maternal death rates had actually risen.[17] Afghanistan's higher rate should not be surprising, since that country has suffered so many years of warfare. Norway's slight rise seems to have been statistically insignificant and its overall rate is still quite low. The maternal death rate in the US, however, seems harder for most people to explain. Don't we spend more per capita on maternity care than any other country in the world? Yes. Don't we apply the highest technology available as often as possible? Yes. The answers to these questions suggest that the challenge of saving mothers' lives requires more than the mere expenditure of resources and the routine use of high technology.

No one can point to any real gain that has come from the increased numbers of surgical births. We can't say, for instance, that it has made birth safer for babies. Credit for the reductions in new-born death rates that have taken place since the seventies belongs to innovations in neonatology, not to higher C-section rates. It's well known that, if anything, higher C-section rates increase the incidence of breathing problems in newborns; they don't reduce them.

What makes the rising C-section rate even more dangerous is that many hospitals discharge women without their first being warned of the symptoms of deep vein thrombosis (DVT)—pain or a hot, swollen place in one of the legs. A DVT can cause a fatal pulmonary embolism or a bowel obstruction (extreme abdominal pain, nausea, and vomiting, and lack of bowel sounds by stethoscope). Both of these potentially fatal complications are related to the damage caused by uterine surgery.[18]

Some women who opt for elective C-sections will inevitably die unnecessarily. The Dutch Maternal Mortality Committee studied just those elective C-sections related to breech that took place between 2000 and 2002, and found that four women died after elective C-sections performed simply because of breech presentation. During that same period, there was no maternal death after an emergency C-section for a breech.[19] These Dutch data undermine the argument that emergency C-sections are necessarily more dangerous for the mother than those that are scheduled.

As I witnessed the maternal death rates rise in the US in the late nineties, and became aware of the degree of underreporting of maternal death rates, I felt that I needed to do something to raise awareness about the effect that the hypermedicalization of birth was having on women and their families. I was inspired by the AIDS Memorial Quilt to create the Safe Motherhood Quilt Project, which is still active today. The AIDS project taught me how powerful it can be for bereaved family and friends to honor and remember people who died from causes that aren't well understood by society in general. It is my hope that the Safe Motherhood Quilt Project will be as effective as the AIDS Memorial Quilt was in identifying a problem that should have national priority and bringing it to the forefront. The goal of the Safe Motherhood Quilt Project is the creation of a comprehensive system to ascertain maternity deaths, coupled with the infrastructure necessary for impartial review by a multidisciplinary team of each and every maternal death that occurs.

The Safe Motherhood Quilt Project has provided me with some insight that has not been generally available. As I see it, the reasons for the increasing death rate of mothers are various, so no simple solution is going to reverse this unacceptable trend. However, one point stands out. The US suffers from a lack of a feedback system, specifically in the area of maternity care, which would allow hospitals and medical professionals who provide such care to see how well they are doing their jobs. Add to this the overuse of technological devices due to fear

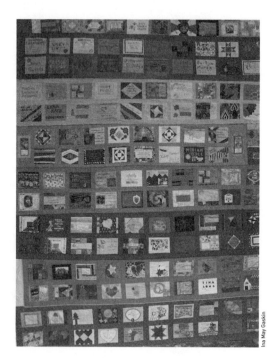

Ina May Gaskin

of malpractice liability, inadequate education of physicians and nurses in time-honored ways of diagnosis or comfort measures, a severe lack of midwives, and poor access to appropriate care early in pregnancy for tens of thousands of low-income women, especially women of color. With our worshipful attitude of high technology as the solution to nearly all problems in the US, our society has too often neglected the all-important human element in maternity care.

LACK OF INFRASTRUCTURE TO COUNT MATERNAL DEATHS

The human rights organization Amnesty International pointed out in a report entitled *Deadly Delivery: The Maternal Health Care Crisis in the USA*, released in 2010, that there is no effective national data gathering effort in the US.[20] In fact, there is such a large degree of underreporting of maternal deaths in the US that the Centers for Disease Control and Prevention (CDC) reported in 1998 that *two-thirds* of the actual deaths that occur could be missing from official reports.[21] There is no strong evidence that this estimate has substantially changed since then.

The reason? Simply put, our data gathering here is extremely haphazard and inconsistent, both on national and state levels. Try this fact, for instance: only six of the fifty states even make it mandatory to report maternal deaths. In other words, in almost every state, it is *optional* for a hospital to report a pregnancy-related death as such and to enter the accurate cause of death on a death certificate. No one at the state or national level has the authority to question this at the time of this writing. The very low importance placed on this important health indicator in the US is illustrated by the fact that the person filling out the death certificate is very often an overtired resident—a doctor in training. Sometimes, it is a clerk who writes in the cause of death on the certificate, someone with no medical training at all and who was not present for any of the dead woman's care. This is simply unacceptable.

The first step in the identification of a maternal death starts with the death certificate and how it is filled out. Maternal deaths are special, because they constitute a subcategory that must be distinguished from the wider category of deaths of women of childbearing age. If they are not distinguished from deaths of women from other causes (for instance, having had a fatal car accident while pregnant), they don't get counted as maternal deaths. The US (and it is the only country I know of that has done this) has produced a standard death certificate form without requiring each state to actually use it. The differences between the various state death certificate forms lie in whether they contain questions related to a deceased woman's pregnancy status within the year prior to her death, and in how these questions, if they exist, are worded. The US Standard Death Certificate has five specific questions designed to elicit the information that analysts need to correctly classify the death as pregnancy-related or not. Death certificates used in some states, however, do not. Should we continue to allow data gathering on a health care issue so important as maternal mortality to be sacrificed to a notion that states' rights are more important than the use of a standard death certificate? I don't think so.

Neither the CDC nor the National Center for Health Statistics has any real authority over how data related to maternal mortality is collected, or any ability to audit the data for accuracy and completeness. The leadership at ACOG has been aware of this situation since at least 1999, so it seems fair to ask why the organization has not used its influence to create the infrastructure that would establish the accountability necessary for any profession involved with life-and-death situations.[22] By contrast, the Royal College of Obstetricians and Gynaecologists (RCOG) in the UK has participated fully in such efforts. I hope to see ACOG follow the good example of RCOG.

Lacking even an accurate count of the maternal deaths that happen, it should come as no surprise to learn that the circumstances surrounding every death are not reviewed by an impartial group (as they are in many other countries, where the idea is to learn from past mistakes, in order to reduce the number of maternal deaths in the future). Fewer than half of the states in the US have any semblance of a maternal mortality and morbidity review committee, according to Amnesty International's *Deadly Delivery* report. Furthermore, US hospitals usually conduct their own reviews following a maternal death, with employees under strict orders not to reveal anything about a death outside a closed-door review meeting. As I write, Congresswoman Lucille Roybal-Allard's MOMS bill, which calls for mandatory maternal mortality and morbidity review in every state (among other important provisions), is making its way through the legislative process. Hopefully, it will be successful.

We also need every state to make it expensive for any person or institution to falsify the information on a death certificate. While I might like to believe that everyone would report everything absolutely accurately in any case that could possibly be a maternal death, my interviews with obstetricians or others who organized or worked on their states' maternal mortality and morbidity review committees tell me otherwise. Here are two sample stories that make my point.

Since I began the Safe Motherhood Quilt Project, I have become the recipient of many reports of maternal deaths. One such report involved a woman whose surviving relative said that her death was caused by a nicked uterine artery during an emergency C-section that reopened after being repaired. In this case, I was able to obtain her death certificate and to read that the "cause of death" box blamed her death on an entirely different cause—amniotic fluid embolism, a cause less likely to be taken as a medical error. Another report was a maternal death that took place in Lee's Summit, Missouri. The woman died because she was married to a man who belonged to a religious cult that taught that wives must be submissive to their husbands, and that seeking medical assistance even in the event of life-threatening complications was a demonstration of a lack of religious faith. In her case, five weeks after nearly a week of labor and the home birth of her stillborn daughter, she died of an untreated infection. According to news reports, the medical examiner and fellow officers urged her husband to give her antibiotics, an action he refused to take. Strangely, the medical examiner who signed her death certificate attributed her death to "natural causes."[23] I am not aware of any other industrialized country in which such deaths can take place, be recorded as due to "natural causes," and instigate no action to prevent more from happening in the future.

Accurate and comprehensive reporting of every maternal death is especially important in a country that has no equivalent of the UK's system of Confidential Enquiries into maternal deaths or the Dutch Maternal Mortality Committee. Every three years, the UK Confidential Enquiries publishes a 300-page report available for sale in bookstores and downloadable in digital form. A chapter is devoted to each of the major causes of maternal death, and citizens and medical professionals in each of the four countries of the UK are able to learn whether there has been improvement or not in the various categories. Besides this, each chapter contains recommendations on how to prevent future maternal deaths, based upon analysis of instances of care found to be substandard.[24] The US should follow the lead of the UK's Confidential Enquiries.

NOTES

1. Gerard G. Nahum, "Predicting Fetal Weight: Are Leopold's Maneuvers Still Worth Teaching to Medical Students and House Staff?" *Journal of Reproductive Medicine* 47 (2002): 271-278.

2. WTVD (Fayetteville, North Carolina), "Doctors Perform C-section on Non-pregnant Woman," April 1, 2010.

3. Murray Enkin, Marc Kierse, James Nielson, Caroline Crowther, Leila Duley, Ellen Hodnett, and Justus Hofmeyr, *A Guide to Effective Care in Pregnancy and Childbirth*, 3rd ed. (New York: Oxford University Press, 2000). Henci Goer's book, *The Thinking Women's Guide to a Better Birth* (New York: Penguin Putnam, 1999), has an excellent discussion of the limitations of EFM.

4. Alice Stewart, Josefine Webb, and David Hewitt, "A Survey of Childhood Malignancies," *British Medical Journal*, June 28, 1958, 1495-1508.

5. J. P. Greenhill, *Obstetrics*, 13th ed. (Philadelphia: W. B. Saunders Company, 1965).

6. H. B. Meier, "The Safety of Diagnostic Ultrasound," *British Journal of Obstetrics and Gynaecology* 94, no. 12 (1987): 1121-1122.

7. Isabel M. Shirley, Fiona Bottomley, and Victor P. Robinson, "Routine Radiographer Screening for Fetal Abnormalities by Ultrasound in an Unselected Low Risk Population," *British Journal of Radiology* 65, no. 775 (1992): 564-569.

8. Marsden Wagner, *Born in the USA: How a Broken Maternity System Must Be Fixed to Put Mothers and Infants First* (Berkeley: University of California Press, 2006).

9. Ibid.

10. L. M. Goetzl, "ACOG Practice Bulletin. Clinical Management Guidelines for Obstetrician-Gynecologists Number 36, July 2002. Obstetric Analgesia and Anesthesia," *Obstetrics and Gynecology* 100, no. 1 (2002): 177-191.

11. M. J. Paech, R. Godkin, and S. Webster, "Complications of Obstetric Epidural Analgesia and Anaesthesia: A Prospective Analysis of 10,995 Cases," *International Journal of Obstetric Anesthesia* 7, no. 1 (1998): 5-11.

12. J. N. Robinson, E. R. Norwitz, A. P. Cohen, T. F. McElrath, and E. S. Lieberman, "Epidural Analgesia and Third- or Fourth-Degree Lacerations in Nulliparas," *Obstetrics and Gynecology* 94, no. 2 (1999): 259-262.

13. See www.rememberthemothers.org.

14. G. J. Barker-Benfield, *The Horror of the Half-Known Life: Male Attitudes toward Women and Sexuality in Nineteenth-Century America* (New York: Routledge, 2000).

15. Nathanael Johnson, "More Women Dying from Pregnancy Complications; State Holds On to Report," *California Watch*, February 2, 2010, http://californiawatch.org/health-and-welfare/more-women-dying-pregnancy-complications-state-holds-report.

16. Mary Beth Pfeiffer, "C-section Rates Tick Upward as Doctors Fear Being Sued," *Poughkeepsie Journal*, May 9, 2010.

17. Margaret C. Hogan, Kyle J. Foreman, Mohsen Naghavi, Stephanie Y. Ahn, Mengru Wang, Susanna M. Makela, Alan D. Lopez, Rafael Lozano, and Christopher J. L. Murray, "Maternal Mortality for 181 Countries, 1980-2008: A Systematic Analysis of Progress towards Millennium Development Goal 5," *The Lancet* 375, no. 9726 (2010):1609-1623, doi:10.1016/S0140-6736(10)60518-1.

18. See www.rememberthemothers.org and the Safe Motherhood Quilt Project for several accounts of such deaths.

19. J. K. Schutte, E. A. Steegers, J. G. Santema, N. W. Schuitemaker, J. van Roosmalen, and the Maternal Mortality Committee of The Netherlands Society of Obstetrics, "Maternal Deaths after Elective Cesarean Section for Breech Presentation in the Netherlands," *Acta Obstetricia et Gynecologica Scandinavia* 86, no. 2 (2007): 240-243.

20. Amnesty International, *Deadly Delivery: The Maternal Health Care Crisis in the USA* (New York: Amnesty International, 2010), www.amnestyusa.org.

21. Centers for Disease Control and Prevention, "Maternal Mortality-United States, 1982-1996," *Morbidity and Mortality Weekly Report* 47, no. 4 (September 4, 1998): 705-707.

22. Timothy Kirn, "Maternal Mortality Rate Grossly Underestimated," *Ob.Gyn. News*, January 11, 2000.

23. KMBC.com, "Family Upset Over Horner's Death Certificate," March 9, 2007, www.kmbc.com/news/11217085/detail.html.

24. Gwyneth Lewis, ed., and The Confidential Enquiry into Maternal and Child Health (CEMACH), *Saving Mothers' Lives: Reviewing Maternal Deaths to Make Motherhood Safer 2003-2005, The Seventh Report on Confidential Enquiries into Maternal Deaths in the United Kingdom* (London: CEMACH, 2007).

BIRTH STORY

Teresa at Home

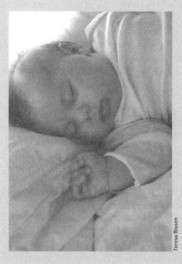

As with many first-time pregnant couples, my husband and I did not decide to pursue a natural birth and, possibly, a home birth until we were well into our first pregnancy. After reading many books, hiring a doula, and attending Bradley classes we became committed to a natural birthing experience, and a home birth intrigued us. However, for our first child, we had to accept a hospital birth. Our OB had a midwife in the practice with whom we felt a strong connection, and although she did home births, she did not offer them to first-time moms. Our goal was to deliver vaginally without medication in the hospital, and to hope for a home birth for future pregnancies.

I was disappointed during my first pregnancy when I was deemed approximately ten days past my due date, and labor was induced with Pitocin. I was informed that my amniotic fluid was low and that "if I did not get induced, the fluid could become so low that an emergency C-section could likely be required." My doctors assured

134

me that induction was my best option, since they "knew I wanted a vaginal delivery." Even though I am a nurse and read as much as I could to avoid induction and unnecessary medical interventions, I felt a bit helpless. Despite my best efforts, when the situation actually arose, I felt I had few options, no words, and no alternatives in my arsenal. I found myself at the mercy of the hospital's policies and protocols—it was more difficult than I imagined to navigate the hospital's labor and delivery system. I felt that my "notions" of a natural delivery were "permitted or tolerated" for a period of time by the medical staff, but eventually they were treated as if they *had* to be abandoned. For every decision and development, I was at odds with specific members of my team and the hospital staff. I knew the kind of reputation I was getting and what the staff was likely saying about me at the desk: "She doesn't want an epidural," "She wants to be disconnected to walk again." When I inquired more about the amniotic fluid levels, I overheard a physician assistant (when talking about me) say, "She's in denial." None of these comments felt conducive to my birthing process or supportive of me.

I ultimately had a vaginal delivery without an epidural. Essentially, for every intervention they suggested, I negotiated for a small walk or allowance to get out of bed. When I was told my water would need to be broken and internal monitoring would be required because I was not progressing (I was stuck at two to three centimeters dilation), I negotiated for thirty minutes to walk around and use the bathroom. During those thirty minutes, I went to the bathroom and my water broke. I stood for as long as I was allowed, leaning on my husband with each contraction. By the time the doctor returned, much to his surprise, I was fully dilated and ready to push. It may sound odd, but once I had my child in my arms, I was celebrating two things: both my delivering a healthy baby boy, and my perseverance to do it vaginally without pain medication. I felt I had secretly succeeded in my quest for a natural delivery. The postdelivery endorphins were absolutely amazing. I remember saying to my husband within an hour of delivering, "Now I know how and why women could have ten to twelve children. When are we doing this again?"

Three years later I became pregnant with our second child. Immediately my husband and I planned for a home birth. We were both excited and nervous about this option. During my seventh month, I stopped my visits to my OB's office and my midwife started home visits. I coasted with absolutely no issues to my due date. Slowly, my due date arrived and passed. Being "overdue" again, at nearly forty-two weeks, became very worrisome to me. I knew that emotional and mental blockages could affect the pregnancy and the birthing process. I had to really sit down and ask myself what, if anything, was preventing me from going into labor, and how to address that. The concerns that weighed heaviest on my mind were the gnawing thoughts in the back of my mind, "What if a home birth is not the best, safest option for me and my infant? What if something goes wrong?" During my daily life as a nurse, I did not advertise my plans for a home birth. I avoided the uncomfortable, unsupportive conversations, telling very few people of our plans. My mother was understandably concerned and not the most supportive of the home birth option we were pursuing. She had *scheduled* a flight for one week after my due date. Surely, I thought, I would have delivered by then. However, it was becoming increasingly clear that my mother would be present for the home birth. Additionally, I was conflicted about purposely planning this birth without her. After all, she had been present for the birth of our son. Having her there but not 100 percent on board was stressful to me; not having planned for her to be there because of her reservations saddened me.

I knew the gnawing thoughts in the back of my mind about the possibly negative outcomes of home birth were unlikely. My pregnancy had been completely healthy and I had delivered vaginally already once before. One thing I was absolutely sure about was that being at odds with the nursery staff after "fighting" for the delivery I desired was definitely something I did not want to endure again unless absolutely necessary. We did not want our baby to be kept away from us and exposed to the nursery if she was born healthy. We wanted her to be with us and nowhere else. This desire overrode any doubts and fears I harbored about a home birth. After several honest conversations with my mother, she was still worried for my health and the baby's health but knew that her visible and verbal support was simply a requirement if she wanted to be present at the birth. When she arrived, and throughout the delivery, her attitude and words were completely supportive. As my pregnancy continued, each night I meditated, telling myself that my body knew what to do (I had done this before!) and talking to my baby, telling her that she was loved, desired, and that we were anxiously awaiting her arrival.

Having previously delivered vaginally with Pitocin, I believed I could handle the painful contractions again. I just had no idea how long it would be this time. (When given Pitocin the first time, I labored for twelve hours total. We could make no predictions about what my body would do without medical intervention.) Having addressed my issues with my mother, the remaining issues centered on the start and end of my labor—when would I begin labor? Could I begin labor? Would my baby be born healthy? With each passing day, I began to doubt my ability to ever go into labor on my own. I was approximately ten days overdue, again. It seemed everyone else's water would "just break" as they were walking down the street. With each morning, I grew more disappointed that I went the entire night without starting labor. It sounds strange when one is nine months pregnant, but I had feelings that I was not a "true woman" because I could not start labor on my own. It became worrisome to me that I would go over my due date by nearly two weeks. How could this happen? Would I need to be induced again after all?

I ultimately went into labor on my own, but with a little help. For my first pregnancy I tried the entire arsenal to start labor, from blue cohosh to castor oil. Nothing worked. I vowed I would not try all of those options again; it was both disappointing and exhausting. After I passed my due date I sought the intervention of my homeopath/osteopath. He gave me several remedies to induce labor. When one of the remedies gave me contractions, the next day we increased its potency. I went to bed that night with some contractions, hoping so much that I would wake up in labor. The clock was ticking on how long I could stay at home before I would need to be admitted for a hospital birth. That night, I woke up at 3:00 AM with consistent contractions. I was ecstatic to be in labor.

I labored for a little over twenty-four hours, with only the last six hours being hard labor. The contractions were five minutes apart all day, thirty to forty-five seconds in length. Consistent enough to be real labor, but too slow to gain real traction. My mother and I cleaned in the morning. I grabbed a nap and went for walks. My doula was with me throughout the day. I sometimes did not believe I was in labor, probably clocking the contractions too often, just to confirm their continued existence. I was partially fearful that if I napped, I would wake up and not be in labor anymore.

Around the twentieth hour of labor, my tolerance of the pain and the fear of how long this could really go on began to get the better of me. I began to doubt my ability to do this, whether I was at home or in the hospital. In all my preparations, I did not mentally prepare for more than twenty hours of labor for my second birth. Both of my labors involved a lot of mind over matter and mantras. I told myself with each contraction that I did not want to go to the hospital because they would make me stay in bed (with this delivery I was keenly aware that lying down not only increased the discomfort, but also slowed down the contractions from five minutes apart to nearly eight minutes apart). I also kept telling myself that if I ended up at the hospital they would likely give me Pitocin. The thought of more painful contractions while being confined to bed was all the motivation I needed to keep going and stay on course for my home birth. Literally, with each wave of each contraction, up until its peak, I would chant silently in my head "I am NOT going to the hospital. I am NOT going to the hospital." (With my first birth, I used the same tactic but my mantra was "I am NOT going to have an epidural. I am NOT going to have an epidural.") Even if I wanted an epidural during the worst of the contractions, when I was not experiencing a contraction, I was adamant I did not want an epidural or, this time, to go to the hospital. Being committed to the birth I wanted each time greatly helped me stay on track. With the contractions I would waiver, but I always came right back to my intentions after their peak. Being at home, relaxed, and able to move about freely at all times was absolutely amazing. No negotiations, no lectures, no monitors. Being surrounded by so many people who fully supported me and my choice of a natural birth undoubtedly assisted in my ability to stay focused. When the contractions were on top of each other I stayed standing up, bending over the back of a large chair. With each of these very strong contractions I imagined the baby coming down the birth canal. This was easier to visualize in the standing position. It felt like everything was in sync. Such visualizations were immensely helpful with each birth. With each contraction I visualized the baby being squeezed and making his or her way down the birth canal. I viewed each contraction as something positive, not negative. With my home birth, I had a great team on board, including my midwife, her assistant, my doula, my mother, and my husband. Each provided outstanding emotional support and I received fabulous, nearly constant back rubs. Being in a conducive environment and knowing that every person present was 100 percent supportive of our process and goals really helped me move past my fears.

I found it very hard to switch gears from contractions to "let's push" in the hospital with my son. In fact, I just really wanted to take a long break! I was unpleasantly surprised with my second birth that I still couldn't switch gears smoothly into pushing. I thought having the prior knowledge of the first pushing session would cure that strange feeling. Unfortunately, it didn't. To be honest, I felt even more nervous when the time to push came for my home birth because of the level of stress and the seriousness of delivering a healthy baby at home. I was on hands and knees, but could not be completely comfortable. I asked my doula to come by my head so I had someone near by. I still did not feel completely comfortable and asked if I could move to my back. It felt much more comfortable to me, even though I knew that being on my hands and knees would create physiological advantages. While lying on my back, I could see everyone's faces and could see and hear the support and excitement from each of them. Everyone had a different level of excitement. I sensed the most nervousness from my mother, and she was nearest to me. I knew where her nervousness was coming from; she would be uneasy until the baby was born healthy. I understood this, as it was part of her role as mother and grandmother. Everyone else on the team provided support of my legs and Janet, my midwife, used her "midwife" voice to focus me. As a nurse, I know that voice well and everything it means. At that moment, I had two omnipresent fears in my mind. First, it was the moment of truth. Months of preparation, worry, love, and excitement were to be answered within minutes. The question of whether I could deliver a healthy baby girl at home would be answered. Second, my thoughts were that I couldn't do this! Again, I didn't think I could push. The support I felt from my team and the voice and words of my midwife focused me on the task at hand. My pushing only lasted for about ten minutes. It was a very stressful, tense ten to fifteen minutes. I focused my efforts by imagining that my healthy baby had traveled her entire journey and that she was ready to emerge. I gained confidence in believing her emergence would be a healthy one.

I know absolutely, without a doubt, that had I not had a scheduled home birth with a midwife that I would not have been allowed to begin my own labor with my second delivery. I would have been induced again. Fortunately, I was off the radar of the medical staff and the antepartum staff. My ultrasound and my fetal non-stress test (NST) were done at a freestanding clinic, to avoid the "you are overdue and you are here, so let's just induce you" conversations. It was such a relief to have that stress removed.

It was absolutely wonderful to deliver at home for the reasons I wanted—for myself and my body. The benefits for my baby daughter were immediately seen also. She was healthy and a happy baby, giving a real smile on her first day of life. She seemed more content than my son was when he was in the hospital. I knew immediately she would not be a fussy baby. I am aware that second-time moms are more relaxed, but I felt that because we were at home and never separated that I could soothe her much more easily than my son. I could distinguish much better between her hunger cries verses her "I am tired" cry.

Since we were at home, we kept having to remind ourselves that she was not three to five days old (as she would have been if we had been admitted to the hospital and then discharged to our home). We had to remind ourselves, more than once, that she was less than twenty-four hours old. The three days that we were at home post-delivery were surreal. We often found ourselves saying, when we were having a wonderful family moment, "If we had delivered in the hospital, we would still be there!" The person who benefited most, and most unexpectedly, from this was my three-and-a-half-year-old son. New York had recently prohibited sibling in-hospital visits, and not being separated from my son greatly assisted in keeping our entire family cohesive, which had a significant impact on his transition to being a big brother.

Having not held my own child or experienced any aspect of motherhood, during my first pregnancy and birth I was focused primarily on my desires for a natural delivery and the intradelivery benefits of a natural delivery for my child. During my second pregnancy, I still had the same focus and intensity in my desire for a vaginal, natural delivery, but I could start to envision the benefits postdelivery for a home birth that did not become clear to me until I had experienced the in-hospital postpartum nursery experience. It wasn't until we experienced it that we fully realized the wonderful benefits to our infant, toddler, and family as a whole that the home birth provided.

—Teresa Bissen

CHAPTER 6

Gathering the Power of Sisterhood

"Sisterhood is powerful" was the most meaningful for me of the feminist slogans heard often during the seventies and eighties. The whole idea of women admiring other women's strength in giving birth had been unexpressed through centuries of US history. Then suddenly, this kind of tribute gained expression in books, poetry, song, art, dance, and storytelling. All of these arts flowed easily from us during the formative years of our midwifery service and the community that surrounded it. It reflected how radical a change it was when my midwifery partners and I decided that we would start trusting each other—and not what we thought of as the medical establishment—when it came to making decisions affecting our bodies and those of our children. There was definitely a feeling of shared strength that went right into the body. During the years of our fastest learning curve, we midwives, in several cases, had the double advantage of attending each other's births. Such experiences knit us very tightly together. Every birth that took place was a learning experience that sent ripples throughout our entire community. Together we learned how to help people negotiate the life passage of birth, and as a few old people came to live among us, we learned about the needs of people and their families as they faced death. Together we learned that the needs around each of these times are similar because of the vulnerabilities that people have during such life passages.

What an exciting life experiment we undertook together. We were a survival show that kept on happening. Every adult was in a position to learn new skills, most of which put us into closer touch with nature. We chopped wood, built fires, and grew food. During the first dozen years or so in our community, most of us had a chance to live in a multifamily dwelling. Each family had its own bedrooms, but the kitchen and the bathroom were shared. (This took compassion, careful planning, good communications skills, and good humor.) Given the close quarters and the common experiences, we shared stories. We talked, and we listened to each other. Spontaneously, we became a childbirth education group by sharing stories of pregnancy and birth. Together we learned how the wide variety of body types and genetic combinations represented in our community all seemed well fitted for survival, at least as concerned the ability to go into labor at the most appropriate time, to labor, to give birth, and to breastfeed. This shared experience gave us great respect for our bodies. Hundreds of us learned that women don't have to carry the kind of fear of birth and of the supposedly ill-designed human female body that has become so widespread in mainstream US culture. We could tell from looking around at each other and knowing each other's birth stories that our bodies were up to the task of giving birth.

Caring for the women in our community also taught me and my partners about the risks posed by certain medical innovations in obstetrical care that we hadn't previously encountered—drugs, for instance, which were widely prescribed before their full range of effects were known. Fortunately, second-wave feminism did inspire a women's health movement that began to research and report on such products as Depo-Provera, a long-acting injectable contraceptive; a drug called diethylstilbestrol (DES, which is discussed in more detail below); and Dalkon Shields and other intrauterine devices (IUDs), to name a few of the so-called innovations. Delving into the literature and relating it to some of our clients who had previously been exposed to some risky products, we soon learned that it was not only the drugs and gynecological implements that we agreed to take and use, but also those that our mothers might have been exposed to that could permanently affect our bodies and our reproductive lives.

DES, THALIDOMIDE, AND GARDASIL: HAVE WE LEARNED YET?

The history of medicine is a saga of episodic progress, of trial frustrated by error, of cruelty mingled with compassion, of devout adherence to ritual alongside ready embrace of innovation, of rejection of discovery alternating with its acclaim.

—Dr. Harold Speert

It was only in the late twentieth century that women began to organize themselves in ways that challenged the near absolute appropriation by the medical profession of how their bodies would be viewed and treated in all aspects of their reproductive lives. Historian Wendy Kline has written a new book about how sisterhood groups in the seventies and eighties organized themselves (and sometimes collapsed in division) in their various attempts to own and redefine how women's bodies are treated in health and in sickness. Her book, *Bodies of Knowledge: Sexuality, Reproduction, and Women's Health in the Second Wave,* presents five case studies in the history of women's health and feminist activism.[1] In well-written, compelling chapters, Kline traces how "difference" feminists, such as the authors of *Our Bodies, Ourselves*—the classic groundbreaking book on women's health that burst upon the scene in 1970—placed the female body at the center of their identity, while "equality" feminists, such as Simone de Beauvoir and Shulamith Firestone, promoted the idea that women could transcend the biological barrier to women's progress only by deemphasizing the female body. Separate chapters examine the genesis of the Boston Women's Health Book Collective and the widespread impact of its work; the groups of women who organized to revolutionize the teaching of pelvic examinations, hoping to eliminate the pain and shame that emanate from the blurred boundaries between sexuality and medicine that provided the background for such exams within the medical context; groups who focused on the difficult and complex issue of pregnancy termination; the strong-minded women who organized to protect their sisters from being unwitting research subjects by publicizing the stories of those who were damaged from having been given Depo-Provera for birth control without informed consent; and the women who pioneered the modern midwifery movement, which sought to create safe spaces in which women could give birth without medical interference unless warranted. Each of the book's chapters contains women's stories of the experiences that drove them to collaborate with other women in order to gain greater knowledge and authority in issues of their reproductive powers, vulnerabilities, and health within a social framework that had barricaded itself for decades from the designs of women—ever since the voices of midwives were silenced.

Kline's book taught me a lot about the struggles and challenges that other women's health activists encountered during the same period of time that my sisters in community and I were organizing ourselves in ways that felt empowering. Like many of the women whose letters or testimony were quoted in her book, I first heard about drugs and treatments that I came to think of as dangerous from stories told by other women. This was the case with diethylstilbestrol (DES), which I became aware of early in my career as a midwife. Because one of the women in our community was a DES daughter (one of an estimated 1.5 million in the US), all of the women living in my community learned how long it could take for negative consequences to become noticeable when a poisonous drug is widely prescribed to pregnant women before adequate research has been done to show that it is harmless. If you were born after 1970, chances are good that you have little awareness about the DES story, so I'll provide a brief summary here. DES is a powerful form of estrogen. The doctor who synthesized it in 1938 started worrying about a possible cancer link only two years later, because he noticed that after powder containing it blew around in his lab, some of the men on his staff who handled it began growing breasts. By this time, though, news of his finding had already created a lot of excitement about the possibilities of its use. Enlisting help from the top animal toxicology and cancer experts in the country, he did his best to dissuade the Food and Drug Administration (FDA) from giving the green light to doctors to prescribe it to women. Despite these efforts, the FDA gave the drug its blessing, and it is estimated that over four million pregnant women in the US were treated with DES between 1941 and 1971 by doctors who believed that it would prevent miscarriage, toxemia, premature birth, overdue birth, unexplained stillbirth, and neonatal death, and ensure the birth of healthy babies. It took thirty years for people to figure out that DES exposure in the womb was causing previously rare vaginal cancers in girls as young as ten, and breast cancer and various vaginal and uterine abnormalities in postpubertal girls—women known today as DES daughters.[2] DES sons, too, were affected, with feminizing effects being reported not just in the first generation, but in the second as well. Studies of third-generation DES exposure are ongoing.

From today's perspective, it is clear that there was a lot of misplaced trust in the wonders of pills prescribed by doctors during the thirty-year period when DES was being prescribed. Women trusted their doctors more than they should have. But what other source of information did they have during a time when so much of the world was still high on the miracles that could be accomplished in laboratories? Who was there to urge caution in adopting too quickly new drugs and treatments designed to improve on nature? Apparently, no one who mattered thought it would be necessary to inform women of the experimental nature of the prescriptions that were being made. Some of the first women who were given DES on an experimental basis were told that the pills were "vitamins."

The first DES study to actually compare outcomes of a group of pregnant women given DES with a group given a placebo took place in the early fifties. It revealed that not only did the women given DES have higher miscarriage rates than those who didn't take the drug, but that none of the other claims of its benefits were true either. Even so, the drug was already too popular with too many influential obstetricians to be stopped by one study showing that it didn't work.[3] History shows us that well-designed studies are often ignored when popular drugs and treatments are involved.

Almost two decades later, the 1971 publication of an article in the *New England Journal of Medicine* detailing several cases of rare vaginal cancers in young women caused the FDA—albeit several months later—to send out a bulletin warning all doctors to stop prescribing DES to pregnant women. According to one of the article's authors, "one of the mothers made an intuitive guess that the cause might be the DES she was given in pregnancy." That caused the researchers who were trying to find the cause of the mysterious cancers that had never been seen before in pubescent girls to add prenatal hormones to the list of questions they were asking the daughters and their mothers. The results of that survey finally revealed DES as the culprit in the cancers.[4]

A similar medical tragedy unfolded in forty-six countries during the late fifties and early sixties. A new drug called thalidomide was sold without prescription to pregnant women with morning sickness and insomnia, causing between ten thousand and twenty thousand babies to be born with severe malformations of their arms and legs. In the case of thalidomide, the drug's effects were noticeable at birth, so the effort to find the cause for the sudden rash of babies born with missing or malformed limbs didn't have to happen more or less by accident, as had been the case with DES.

With this history to ignite them, the women's health movement of the seventies grew as a response to the dangerous lack of research required before drugs were marketed and prescribed to women. Barbara Seaman, a pioneer of that movement, originally became involved because her doctor prescribed her a drug while she was lactating that could have killed her newborn son. "He recovered, but in one sense I did not, for I would never again trust a doctor blindly," Seaman wrote in *The Greatest Experiment Ever Performed on Women.* She helped found a campaign demanding research into the birth control pill (at the time of its release, birth control was ten times more powerful and more likely to cause fatal blood clots or other adverse effects than present formulas, which are still not free of these side effects), and succeeded in having the first warning label put on a drug, so that patients could be informed of the hazards of drugs prescribed to them.

Given the amount of suffering caused by the twin tragedies of DES and thalidomide not so many decades ago, and the incredible steps forward initiated by certain insightful feminists of the seventies, you might suppose that there would be a heightened sense of awareness about the dangers of rapid adoption of new medications or techniques in maternity wards. However, the trend has gone astonishingly far in the opposite direction. When we take a look at the current state of women's health and maternity care in the US, it is clear that it is even more necessary than ever for a renewed women's health movement to emerge, and to keep constantly vigilant and skeptical with regard to new drugs that may be prescribed to women or their children. Take the case of Gardasil. This vaccine began being heavily marketed in 2006 in the mass media as effective for the prevention of four human papilloma viruses (HPV) in teenage girls. With about 70 percent of cases of cervical cancers involving previous infection with HPV (commonly known as genital warts), the claim has been that three doses of the vaccine would significantly reduce a teenage girl's chance of contracting cervical cancer later in life. How quickly medical professionals and the general public forgot (or never learned) the lessons that should have been absorbed from the drug fiascos of the sixties and seventies. Slightly more than six thousand women between the ages of sixteen and twenty-six were given the drug in trials before it went on the market in 2006. Obstetricians and pediatricians were urged to prescribe the vaccine to girls as young as eleven, the idea being to vaccinate them before they might engage in sexual activity and possibly contract HPV. Many doctors made sure that their own daughters were vaccinated.

It didn't take long before reports of adverse events following injection with Gardasil began being reported to the Food and Drug Administration. By May 31, 2010, more than sixteen thousand adverse events had been reported, along with fifty-three deaths in the US (twenty-nine of which have been confirmed by the FDA). There have been reports of fainting, headache, extreme muscle weakness, dizziness, muscle pain, seizures, hair loss, heart palpitations, spells of blindness, and joint tenderness. In spite of these reports, the Centers for Disease Control and Prevention and the FDA consider Gardasil "safe and effective." Gardasil continues to be prescribed to young women, even though it will be decades before a large enough number of teenage girls reach the age when women are most likely to contract cervical cancer. Only then will it be known if Gardasil really lives up to the claims made by its manufacturer.[5]

MENSTRUATION-SUPPRESSING DRUGS

Near the end of the twentieth century, pharmaceutical companies apparently decided that the time was ripe for profits to be made by manipulating women who dislike having periods. Because probably a majority of US women by this time had little fear of modifying their hormones, all they had to do was promise fewer and lighter periods— even as cancer rates continued their upward climb, and uncounted numbers of women continued to die each year from strokes and blood clots that stemmed from their use of various hormonal contraceptive products. The market for menstruation-suppressing drugs was $2.2 billion in 2003, the year that Dr. Susan Rako's book, *No More Periods?*

The Risks of Menstrual Suppression and Other Cutting-Edge Issues About Hormones and Women's Health, was published. Her view that "[m]anipulating women's hormonal chemistry for the purpose of menstrual suppression threatens to be the largest uncontrolled experiment in the history of medical science," is one that many women are still in denial about, but there are signs that such attitudes are beginning to shift, possibly because of the number of alarming side effects being reported at such sites as www.askapatient.com. Keep in mind that no one has any idea of long-term risks.

Dr. Rako's book is one of the only contemporary sources available to women that provides information about the risks that come along with hormone tampering. Given the number of women who have no idea of the potential danger that drastically altering their hormones can pose and who also hate their periods, I recommend it as a necessary antidote to the constant television advertising that makes menstrual suppression so attractive to young women who have little access to other views related to women's health. Warnings on the internet about serious side effects such as, "abdominal pain, chest pain, heavy bleeding, eyesight or vision changes, or severe leg pain," make it obvious that these drugs have had dire consequences for women. How sad that we have no one of the caliber of Dr. Frances Kelsey and Dr. David Kessler at the FDA at the time that I write.

TOLERANCE FOR ELECTIVE SURGERY

In recent years, women's health advocates have had to weigh in on the debate surrounding breast implants. Since the nineties, my midwifery partners and I have encountered an increasing number of women who have undergone elective breast surgery. Unless we are talking about necessary mastectomy for cancer, most breast surgery is elective—that is, the woman would survive without it. The usual story with the women we meet who underwent breast reduction surgery in particular is that they chose to have it when they were too young to realize that they might want to maintain a maximal ability to breastfeed a baby later in life. Women under the age of twenty usually can't imagine how they'll feel later in life, if and when they are struck by the urge to have a baby. While it is true that some women are able to breastfeed after such surgery, those who had too much milk-producing tissue removed or whose nipples were excised and relocated to a more central point on the smaller breast may not be able to make enough milk to sustain a baby or to move milk out of the breast at all. Whenever I meet a woman who now regrets having sought out or agreed to such surgery, I am reminded how far increasing numbers of doctors, especially surgeons, have deviated from the Hippocratic Oath to first do no harm.

Every young woman in our culture has to come to terms with the size of her breasts. Breasts are fetishized in our culture, so, for a lot of women, they assume a greater importance than any part of the body. Girls with small breasts are often teased by classmates and made to feel unattractive—the way I often felt when I was growing up. In those days, small-breasted girls used to wad up toilet paper and stuff it into their bras. I never tried that myself; my way to avoid being teased was to hunch my shoulders forward, hoping that no one would notice my chest. I carried myself that way until I was in my late twenties, when I finally began to walk with a full sense of gratitude for my healthy body. Remembering my early years, I do understand how easy it can be to exploit the insecurities US women often develop about their breasts. It's often hard for a young woman to know that while the looks of breasts seem to matter most when she hasn't had them that long, the way they *feel* is going to matter a lot more as life goes on.

Breast implants are sold as "prosthetics" (albeit the kind that must be replaced every few years) that are advertised to cure low self-esteem in women. At the same time, at least seven different studies have shown that women who had implants are three times more likely to commit suicide than women without them. The suicide rate increases to six times more likely when twenty years have passed since the first surgery.[6] It's possible, of course, that women who are already quite depressed are more likely than others to choose breast implant surgery, but don't we have to wonder how many became depressed when they realized that their subsequent illnesses were caused by breast implants whose risks were unknown to them? Whatever is the case, more than 300,000 US women chose to have breast augmentation surgery in 2007, according to the American Society of Plastic Surgery. That's a lot of elective surgery.

Regulations surrounding elective breast surgery have been almost nonexistent. Most of the women who choose it are probably unaware that *anyone* with an MD can legally perform breast implant surgery in a doctor's office in most of the US. No specialized training is required; one can be a podiatrist, an obstetrician, a psychiatrist, or a pediatrician and still be within the law in carrying on a practice in the lucrative plastic surgery business. Early in 2010, an Atlanta opthalmologist, Dr. Rajeesh Rangaraj, had to call the emergency operator when a breast implant patient nearly bled to death in his office during surgery. The woman, Kenyatta Brown, was awake, as she was under only a local anesthetic, so she heard and still remembers the panicked phone call describing how blood was spurting uncontrollably from her wound.[7] A fast ambulance ride to a hospital and quick attention from a surgical team were necessary to save her life. Was she the first woman to experience a life-threatening complication during breast implant surgery? The answer is no, but getting solid information on what the toll of near-misses and deaths associated with implant surgery has been is far from easy. Dr. Frank B. Vasey, one of the leading experts in the US on complications following breast implant surgery, mentioned in an editorial in a rheumatology journal a Pittsburgh woman who developed an acute illness suggesting toxic shock immediately after implant placement in 1979. Infection was ruled out, but she had to have her silicone breast implants removed ten days after placement, after which she made a complete recovery.[8] Every now and then a woman who had a life-threatening complication reveals her story, such as the woman who suffered toxic shock after her implant operation and suffered the amputation of her feet and fingers.[9]

Most US women are unlikely to know that medical opinion on the safety of breast implants varies greatly, depending upon the specialty of the doctor one asks. In general, it is safe to say that surgeons have far fewer worries about the safety of breast implants than do rheumatologists or other internists, the doctors who are most likely to provide care for women exhibiting symptoms after having implants. Dr. Vasey points out in his important book *The Silicone Breast Implant Controversy: What Women Need to Know* that surgeons tend to focus on a single problem or area of the body. They deal with a specific surgical problem, perform the surgery, and then they are finished, provided there are no immediate complications. If medical problems occur after incisions heal, a surgeon will usually refer the patient to an internist, a rheumatologist, or a family physician. Rheumatologists and other internists, therefore, are more apt to develop an interest in silicone disease than are surgeons. To those internists who become expert in this area and see hundreds of women with the same problems, Dr. Vasey explains, "The constellation of silicone-induced signs and symptoms soon becomes clear."[10] They often observe that when implants are removed from women who are experiencing complications in their immune system, their symptoms usually improve and sometimes disappear entirely. This suggests a link between breast implants and autoimmune disorders.

When foreign material finds its way into human tissue, its presence causes the body's immune system to try to fight it off as an army might fight off an invader. The larger the surface area of the foreign material, the larger the response from the immune system is. Even so-called saline implants, which were marketed after the initial fears about silicone gel breast implants were widely publicized, are silicone bags containing salty water and are thus likely to provoke the same sort of response that has been reported with silicone gel implants. The manufacturers of the newest generation of silicone gel implants admit on their websites that these "are not lifetime devices" and that "silent ruptures" may occur. Because of these problems, they recommend that every woman with an implant have regular MRIs every two years to detect this kind of rupture and the resulting silicone that seeps into the body. When silent ruptures are found, removal of the implants is imperative. However, surgery of this kind is rarely covered by women's insurance policies, and neither are the MRIs.

And what are the autoimmune disorders that have been reported after breast implants are placed? The list of symptoms commonly reported is long and varied: swelling of lymph nodes, extreme pain in muscles and joints, chronic fatigue that can't be relieved by sleep, memory loss, difficulty in swallowing, numbness, hardening and tightening of the skin, dry eyes, shortness of breath, and loss of sex drive are some examples. Many women have several symptoms simultaneously. Such symptoms often take more than five years to show up after silicone is installed in the body. Autoimmune diseases that may be directly related to, or worsened by, silicone exposure include rheumatoid arthritis, scleroderma, systemic lupus erythematosus, fibromyalgia, multiple sclerosis (MS), amyotrophic lateral sclerosis (ALS), silicone-associated connective tissue disorder, and dermatomyositis. The problem facing internists is that burden of proof seems to have been placed on them, and they are faced with a comparatively new disease category: silicone-related immune disorders. The lack of coverage in the mainstream media of the autoimmune disorders following implants that tens of thousands of women have reported to rheumatologists since the eighties has continued to encourage a false sense of security and makes it easy for women to believe that breast implant complications are rare, minor, and nothing to worry about.

Constant media promotion of breast implants has taught women not to fear this kind of surgery, and this has been especially true since the turn of the century. The fact that implant surgery can be legally performed in a doctor's office tells women that this is a simple, rather routine operation. However, most women don't know that a "grandfathering" loophole in the FDA existed in the seventies, and this allowed breast implant manufacturers to escape any requirement to provide additional safety data about their products. During the nineties, many women came forward and claimed that serious health problems they experienced after their implants were installed had to be related to the presence of silicone in their bodies. The FDA seemed to be on the right track in early 1992, when Commissioner Dr. David Kessler, to his great credit, made the following statement: "The burden of proof is an affirmative one, and it rests with the manufacturer. We know more about the life span of automobile tires than we do about the longevity of breast implants."[11] Kessler was responding to the many reports of ruptured implants that spilled silicone into the bodies of women who had no idea this could happen. Photos of breasts containing implants that had hardened into what looked like tennis balls and migrated sideways or downward were included in some of the television reports on implant disasters. Whatever their complaints, enough women came forward during that time that by 2003, Dow Corning had quietly released settlement packages to distribute 4.6 billion dollars to injured women, and several other manufacturers, including Bristol-Myers Squibb, 3M, and Baxter, had also offered sizeable settlements.[12] Is it possible to believe that those corporations would have spent all that money if they hadn't thought that silicone leaking into women's bodies might be the cause of the women's illnesses?

Despite the huge numbers of women with breast implants who have yet to give birth, there has been very little curiosity on the part of company researchers about the effects on babies of breast milk containing silicone and platinum salts. Platinum, by the way, is added to silicone by some implant manufacturers to create a gel. Both substances have been found in the milk of women with silicone gel implants, and nature didn't mean for either of them to be there. Mentor, the manufacturer of several FDA-approved implants, apparently wants us to feel better about having such materials in our bodies when it publishes statements such as these on its website: "Silicone is derived from silicon, a semi-metallic or metal-like element that in nature combines with oxygen to form silicon dioxide, or silica. Beach sand, crystals, and quartz are silica. Silica is the most common substance on earth." Well, yes, but that doesn't mean that it's good to put it into the body or that it would be good for babies to eat it.

The same website provides this answer to the question about the possibility of developing "allergies" to silicone in the body: "It is possible for anyone to develop an allergy to almost any substance on earth, however silicone allergies are very rare. We are all exposed to silicone in our environment everyday. It is found in many household items, such as polishes, suntan and hand lotion, antiperspirants, soaps, processed foods, waterproof coatings, and chewing gum." Again, there are several items on that list that I wouldn't want to eat or have surgically implanted into my body.

The website's answer to the important question of whether babies might be harmed by milk from mother's breasts that contain implants was this: "There have been concerns raised regarding potential damaging effects on children born of mothers with breast implants. A review of the published literature suggests that the information is insufficient to show definitive conclusions." So much for the babies.

Another statement on the website is noteworthy for its lack of clarity: "Although there are no current methods for detecting silicone levels in breast milk, a study measuring silicon (one component in silicone) levels did not indicate higher levels in breast milk from women with silicone-filled gel implants when compared to women without implants."[13] When I was an English teacher, I would mark a sentence like that one as unacceptable, because it contradicts itself.

Two researchers did report on a small number of cases in the *Journal of the American Medical Association* in 1994, a report in which they "demonstrated sclerodermalike esophageal dysmotility (difficulty in swallowing) in children breast-fed by mothers with silicone breast implants."[14] We're still waiting for a larger study, preferably one funded by a nonprofit, impartial group of scientists with experience in toxicology. Although many children breast-fed on breasts with implants have displayed no harmful effects, some parents have claimed that their children have suffered bad effects. One such mother, a blogger, wrote: "I had silicone implants when I breastfed my infant daughter 15 years ago, and since then, she has suffered all sorts of strange illnesses, with some symptoms very similar to my own from my silicone poisoning."[15]

I still find it hard to swallow the claim that silicone-laced milk should be considered harmless until proven guilty when ingested by the most vulnerable humans on the planet, since allowing them to drink even teensy amounts is completely experimental. I wish that researchers today were like Dr. James Simpson and his colleagues back in the mid-nineteenth century, who used themselves as guinea pigs when they wanted to learn about the effects of chloroform used as an anesthetic. Would researchers today agree to ingest amounts of silicone and platinum (in levels comparable to those that babies might receive in breast milk) to see how they fare (remembering that breast-fed babies ordinarily have no other source of food for the first several months)? That would be an interesting study, but it's obviously not going to happen.

In 2005, the FDA—by this time, Dr. Kessler was no longer commissioner—assembled a panel of doctors, psychologists, and representatives from Mentor, the manufacturer of two silicone gel implants, to decide if their new, "improved" silicone gel implants were improved enough to be approved by the FDA. I would recommend that anyone considering breast implantation surgery first read the transcribed notes of this FDA meeting.[16] Except for a dermatologist and a psychiatrist, every doctor who was chosen to be a voting member of the panel was a surgeon. Not a single internist, family physician, pediatrician, or rheumatologist was included, which may be the reason why so little attention was given to data about serious autoimmune disorders that have been linked to various kinds of implants since they first appeared on the market. Whoever decided who would be included as voting members on the panel had already decided to ignore the many case reports of postimplant patients' complaints of multiple symptoms, and to give Mentor implants the benefit of the doubt. One voting member asked what effect escaped silicone might have on the breast milk ingested by babies, but got no answer from the Mentor representative, who could only say that animal studies could possibly be done, but that even those results might not apply to humans.

Never before reading the notes of the FDA meeting had I realized that there were measurement systems such as the "Sexual Attractiveness Scale," the "Tennessee Self-Concept Scale," and the "Rosenberg Self-Esteem Scale." One industry representative referred to a study of women who claimed that their implants had given them "improved sexual satisfaction." A couple of panel members wanted to know about the strength of the studies carried out by the manufacturers, and were told that the manufacturers didn't keep track of the women who decided to have their implants removed within a period of two to three years after installation. One way of sweetening the results in a "study" is to exclude possible problems in the study design itself.

Near the end of the meeting, one of the voting members, Dr. Newburger, the dermatologist, remarked: "I don't have a good sense, other than increasing chest size, that this [the new silicone gel implant] really is all that effective." Only one other voting member agreed with her and voted against approval.

Just before the vote, several members of the public were permitted to speak. Those who spoke against approval of the new implants spoke early: a representative from the National Women's Health Network and a woman with a master's degree in public health both pointed to the inadequacy of the statistics presented by the Mentor representatives. Only one other public representative spoke against approval, and she, too, spoke early—her mother had had silicone gel implants installed after a double mastectomy, experienced numerous complications and illnesses thereafter, and, after ten years of constantly deteriorating health, committed suicide. Seven women spoke in favor of approval. Three were sisters who had all undergone mastectomies because they had several relatives who had died from breast cancer. One was a plastic surgeon who reported that she performed four hundred to five hundred breast implant surgeries per year. Another was the president of an association of plastic surgery nurses, who pooh-poohed what she called the "mass hysteria" that the FDA had caused when it put a moratorium on silicone gel implants during the nineties. She remarked that the FDA did not keep people from smoking cigarettes, in spite of their "known destructive side effects," implying that the same lack of regulation should be applied to breast implants.

Just before the vote was taken, each member was asked to make a brief statement. One who voted against approval reminded the others that implants would surely be put into hundreds of thousands of women, that silicone gel implants had a thirty-year "checkered history," and that the Mentor implant was still too new to have been well evaluated. On the other hand, Barbara Manno, who holds a PhD in pharmacology and toxicology, worried about the possibility of the FDA panel stepping too much on the company's toes. "Given the testimony here, etcetera, from the public and what I heard from the public the last time," she said, "if the doctors and the company provide the information, I think we have got enough to approve this and that the recipients of the device will have a choice. And it isn't to have a choice, they can make a choice and it's tough luck if it doesn't work. No, I don't mean that. I would like that stricken. No, I believe it will work, I think, based on what I have seen here and, please, I did not mean that the way it sounded."[17]

The vote to approve the Mentor implants was seven to two.

THE ELECTIVE C-SECTION FAD

As described earlier, at the time of this writing, the US national cesarean rate is more than six times what it was in 1968, when it was 5 percent of all births.

Back in 1979 when this had first become a concern, a report was commissioned by the Department of Health, Education, and Welfare to evaluate what was happening with the sharp increase in the C-section rate, which quadrupled between 1968 and 1980. Its findings? The most frequent reason given by more than one hundred physicians interviewed by the analyst who authored the report was fear of a malpractice suit if a C-section was not performed. The analyst observed: "Although physicians freely agreed 'off the record' that fear of a suit prompted Caesareans and that this was commonly discussed, few actually knew of a colleague who had been sued." (Remember: this research was done in the seventies, when malpractice lawsuits were still relatively rare). The next most frequent cause for the increase in the rate of surgery was the policy that once a woman had a C-section, she had forever lost her chance to give birth vaginally. Women in the eighties rebelled against this policy by joining the vaginal birth after cesarean (VBAC) movement, whether that meant finding a physician or midwife to assist such a birth or giving birth at home without professional assistance. The third most mentioned cause for the increase in the C-section rate had to do with physician training. Physicians gave many examples of how much their training concentrated on using electronic fetal monitoring, ultrasonography, and fetal scalp sampling and how little training they got in basic obstetrical skills such as monitoring the fetal heart with a stethoscope, manually changing a baby's position in the uterus, conducting a breech birth, and manually assessing mothers' pelvic size relative to the size of their babies.[18]

In 1985, the *New England Journal of Medicine* published that era's equivalent of Dr. DeLee's 1920 recommendation that all babies be pulled from their mothers' bodies with forceps: the 1985 article recommended that all pregnant women should be required to have "prophylactic" C-sections and that those who chose to refuse should have to sign a consent form for the attempt at vaginal delivery.[19]

In the late nineties, W. Benson Harer Jr., former president of the ACOG, gave further support to the extreme position that elective C-sections were superior to vaginal birth when he began doing interviews on radio and television in which he suggested that an elective C-section might be the best way to avoid bodily harm caused by vaginal birth. "For the mother, it reduces the damage to the pelvic structures which would lead to urinary or fecal incontinence," he told the *Boston Globe*. "And, for the [full-term] baby, an elective C-section is probably as safe or maybe even safer than attempting a vaginal delivery."[20] Harer's speaking campaign, which went on for a few years after his presidency at ACOG was over, neglected to mention that even a scheduled C-section, with no emergency, has an almost three times greater chance than vaginal birth of resulting in the woman's death. There was, of course, no mention either of the increased rate of postbirth infections, potentially fatal pulmonary embolisms, and risks to future pregnancies caused by the greatly increased rate of surgical births.[21]

Obstetricians who disagreed with Harer were able to air their views in publications read by other doctors, but the mainstream media didn't see the need to provide such balance. Apparently, if a doctor said it, it must be right, even if his colleagues challenged his views. "Patients are being hoodwinked into choosing cesareans by overblown fears of incontinence and other risks associated with trial by labor," said Dr.

Robert K. DeMott, chief of staff at Bellin Memorial Hospital in Green Bay, Wisconsin. "Putting it bluntly," he said, "it's unethical to recommend a practice that leads to more patient deaths."[22]

The many women who believed Dr. Harer's scary thoughts about their pelvic structures—thoughts that were thrown out so casually during his breakfast talk show appearances—must have assumed that most older women (who gave birth the old way) were quietly wearing adult diapers. Too bad more women didn't get to hear about Dr. DeMott's views.

ORGANIZING TO IMPROVE THE LOT OF MOTHERS

It has been a long time since any national energy was expended to improve the status of mothers in the US, but the time to reverse the current situation is clearly here. Since we find ourselves with a rising maternal death rate despite our spending more per capita on maternity care than any other nation in the world, it is clear that we are doing something wrong. Most likely, we are doing a lot of things wrong. How do we identify and prioritize these things?

Let's face it. We're not going to know exactly what to do about our predicament unless we start by creating the infrastructure that most of us probably think we already have in place. If we don't do this, we shall condemn ourselves and future generations to guessing the causes for the rising maternal mortality rate. That will get us nowhere. Unless we take the trouble to collect good data, we won't know for a fact what is causing the rising maternal mortality rate. Without the facts, women, midwives, and home birth will continue to be made the scapegoats for whatever is wrong with maternity care in the US, and we will not solve our problems.

It's time to organize to create the pressure necessary to force the establishment of a national system of data collection of information related to maternal death. Let's start pressuring state legislatures to pass laws that require accuracy of counting, and to create mortality and morbidity review committees in every state. In the states in which such a committee already exists but issues no public report of its findings, this lack should be addressed.

I am optimistic about the possibility of women today organizing themselves sufficiently to push for the creation of public policy that would positively affect the status of motherhood. Generally, when Internet discussions about childbirth issues come up, an argument develops between the side that favors a more medicalized approach to birth and one that favors a less interventive approach. We all know how polarized arguments can get about whether all pregnancies should be continued or not, where babies should be born, and how babies should be fed. Adopting the goal of fixing the maternal death data collection system in our country would be one that could pull together women who may disagree with each other on other issues. How could anyone defend a position that it is too much work and expense for our country to accurately count maternal deaths?

NOTES

1. Wendy Kline, *Bodies of Knowledge: Sexuality, Reproduction, and Women's Health in the Second Wave* (Chicago: The University of Chicago Press, 2010).
2. Barbara Seaman, *The Greatest Experiment Ever Performed on Women: Exploding the Estrogen Myth* (New York: Seven Stories Press, 2003).
3. Barbara Seaman and Gideon Seaman, *Women and the Crisis in Sex Hormones* (New York: Rawson Associates Publishers, Inc., 1977).
4. Arthur Herbst, H. Ulfelder, and D. C. Poskanzer, "Adenocarcinoma of the Vagina: Association of Maternal Stilbestrol Therapy with Tumor Appearance in Young Women, *New England Journal of Medicine* 284, no. 15 (1971): 878-881.
5. Sharyl Attkisson, "Vaccine Watch: Gardasil Side-Effect," CBS News, July 8, 2008, http://www.cbsnews.com/8301-500803_162-4240888-500803.html.
6. Anita Manning, "Breast Implants Linked to Higher Suicide Rates," *USA Today*, April 6, 2007.
7. Colin Stewart, "Lessons of 3 Breast Implant Disasters," *Orange County Register*, July 19, 2010.
8. Frank B. Vasey, S. Alireza Zarabadi, Mitchell Seleznick, and Louis Ricca, "Where There's Smoke, There's Fire: The Silicone Breast Implant Controversy Continues to Flicker: A New Disease that Needs to be Defined," *The Journal of Rheumatology* 30, no, 10 (2003): 2092-2094, accessed at http://www.breastimplantinfo.org/what_know/controversy.html.
9. *The Sun Magazine*, Letters, September 2010, 13-14.
10. Frank B. Vasey, *The Silicone Breast Implant Controversy: What Women Need to Know* (Freedom, California: The Crossing Press, 1993).

11. Ibid.
12. Vasey et al., "Where There's Smoke, There's Fire."
13. www.mentorwwllc.com.
14. J. J. Levine and N. T. Ilowite, "Sclerodermalike Esophageal Disease in Children Breast-fed by Mothers with Silicone Breast Implants," *Journal of the American Medical Association* 271, no. 3 (1994): 213-216.
15. http://beautyandthebreast.org.
16. http://www.fda.gov/ohrms/dockets/ac/05/transcripts/2005-4101t3.htm.
17. Ibid.
18. Helen Marieskind, *An Evaluation of Caesarean Section in the United States: Executive Summary*(Washington DC: US Department of Health, Education, and Welfare, 1979).
19. G. Feldman and J. Freiman, "Prophylactic Cesarean Section at Term?" *New England Journal of Medicine* 312, no. 19 (1985): 1264-1267.
20. Michael Lasalandra, "C-sections on Demand are Rising Fast," *Boston Globe*, April 20, 2004.
21. M. Hall and S. Bewley, "Maternal Mortality and Mode of Delivery," *Lancet* 354 (1999): 776.
22. Greg Borzo, "Elective C-sections Stir up Controversy," *Ob.Gyn. News*, October 1, 2000.

What's a Father-to-Be to Do?

I help men do what they don't want to do so they can achieve
what they want to achieve.

—John Wooden, UCLA basketball coach

What does a man want to achieve when it comes to birth? What he generally wants is safe passage through the various unknowns presented by pregnancy, labor, and birth (let's call these the "foothills"), so that he can get to the "summit": the enjoyment of living up to his own expectations in raising his family. Now if he has been well exposed to the dominant mindset of fear of birth in our culture (as have most men), he worries about his partner and his baby and how he can help them escape all the scary "what if" scenarios that have probably gone through his mind since he learned about the pregnancy. He generally has strong urges to be protective and may have little or no idea of how to act on these urges. My aim in this chapter is to give some idea of how to channel this sort of energy.

Laboring women aren't the only ones going through a deep transformation when a baby is born. Babies' fathers also go through powerful inner changes as well—especially when they are ready to be as close to their partners as possible during the process. Fathers of earlier generations, when they were still prevented from being with their wives during labor and birth, were less likely to feel comfortable about holding their newborn babies and participating in their early care than I observe men to be when they have been closely involved during labor and birth. Physically separated from both their wives and their babies for the first several days following birth, fathers in the past were insulated to a great degree from the realities of how babies are born. With their experience of becoming a parent already at a remove because of biology (fathers do not feel the growing fetus in their own bodies), the consequences of this kind of separation during and after birth can be enormous. When modifications in hospital practice began to take place in the early seventies, researchers noted that fathers who were present when their babies were born and had early physical contact with the babies were much more likely to cuddle their newly born babies, to talk or sing to them, and to be skilled at calming them than fathers who had had no such contact.

Fathers who are present when their babies are born seem to derive an increased respect for their partners from the experience. The same goes for their perceptions of the abilities of their newborns. Fathers are often just as surprised as are the mothers when the baby, placed face down on the mother's belly, begins to crawl toward her breast. They are impressed not only by the ability to crawl but also by the baby's knowledge of where to go and how hard the baby struggles (without complaint) to get there.

One of my favorite stories about a new father discovering fathering skills came from a lactation consultant friend of mine. This particular baby was two days old, quite fussy, and hadn't yet managed to get a good latch onto her mother's breast. According to my friend, the mother was beginning to become frustrated enough to consider giving up on breast-feeding. At that point, her husband (who cared for a few goats in his spare time) stepped in and saved the day. Cuddling his newborn daughter to his chest—as he later explained to my friend—he began to experience an impulse to lick her, in the way he had often seen nanny goats licking their newborns. (Never before could he have imagined himself doing such a thing.) At any rate, he decided to follow that impulse and began to lick his daughter's soft cheek and forehead. The effect upon her was dramatic: her crying stopped, and as she calmed down, she began to open her mouth in the unmistakable ways babies do when they are most ready to take the breast. Now she was ready for her mother, and she went to her breast and latched on without further ado.

I believe the four key concepts regarding labor and birth for fathers-to-be to keep in mind are these: (1) know the basics of sphincter law; (2) know how to keep your partner's oxytocin and beta-endorphin levels as high as possible and her adrenaline levels low; (3) she leads, you follow; and (4) have trust in her monkey self.

SPHINCTER LAW

Any woman who has pushed a baby out without any pain-numbing medication will say that the sensation feels just like having to poop something really big and hard. Enough women manage to go through an entire pregnancy without realizing that they are pregnant that we now have a television documentary series devoted to interviewing these women and presenting reenactments of what happened. It's hard for most women who have been pregnant to imagine that this is possible, but it does happen more often than most realize. The common thread in these cases is that the women go into labor but don't realize that it's labor. They experience pain that comes in waves, but they describe it as like a stomach flu or severe constipation. Occasionally, the woman thinks she might have a ruptured appendix, and in these cases, she goes to a hospital emergency room. The women, of course, are laboring without medication or preconceptions about what they should be feeling. Typically, those who interpret their sensations as signs of constipation just move around a lot and eventually sit on the toilet, hoping to finally relieve themselves, and yes, sometimes the baby falls into the toilet and is none the worse for it except for having a hard-to-explain birth story (if the parents decide to share the story with the world).

One way you can help your partner during pregnancy is to let her know that you are not horrified (or even turned off) by the idea of her pooping. (If you are now, get over it. This change is possible.) She manages to deal with the fact that you do, so fair's fair—right? Since I have met a few couples whose agreement before meeting me was apparently that each had to leave the room if the urge to fart came (just imagine how this can interfere with the woman's sensations as she begins to push her baby out), I try to address this problem during pregnancy. While in Austria a few years ago, I found a children's book with an eye-catching title, which I'll translate literally: *The Little Mole Who Wanted to Know Who Pooped on His Head*. Translations of this extremely popular book have appeared all over the world, so you can find it in English, but the American English translation of the title has been made euphemistic: *The Little Mole Who Went in Search of Whodunit*. Before you decide that my weirdness in suggesting that you buy your partner this book is too much, listen to the practical reasons for it. First, it will demonstrate how comfortable you suddenly have become about your partner's bodily functions. Second, it will introduce a kind of humor that may have been lacking in your relationship up to this point. The good thing about this is that such humor may greatly help your partner get over any hang-ups about poop that she may have (which can interfere more than you might imagine with her ability to give birth vaginally). Enjoy the silly, childish humor. This can come in handy not only during labor but when the two of you are dealing with the poop that your baby will give you.

OXYTOCIN HIGH, ADRENALINE LOW

Just to be clear, I must specify that we're talking about endogenous oxytocin—the kind that is produced by the body—rather than the synthesized kind that is brought into the body via an intravenous line. Its benefits are that high levels of oxytocin help to keep effective contractions of the uterus happening. Oxytocin levels rise when the woman is feeling happy, grateful, amused, praised, or loved, so anything you say or do to elicit any of these emotional responses should be helpful. Don't worry about her getting bored with how often you tell her that you love or appreciate her. The wonderful thing about keeping oxytocin levels high is that when this is achieved, adrenaline levels tend to stay low. This is because oxytocin and adrenaline are antagonistic to each other—in other words, when one is high, the other is low.

High adrenaline levels also have an emotional component: they rise when the woman is fearful, angry, or otherwise stressed. Of course, you won't want to be the one to cause any of these emotional states. One thing you should imprint on your memory: never, never ask a laboring woman how she is feeling while she is in the middle of a contraction.

SHE LEADS, YOU FOLLOW

Think of labor as a dance and that your partner is the one who leads how the two of you will move through the dance. You'll learn quickly how to follow her cues if you are observant. That's pretty simple, isn't it? You can practice while she is still pregnant.

I remember one conscientious father-to-be who would have been happy if his wife had enjoyed staring into his eyes throughout labor (as she did for maybe half an hour). At length, though, she made it clear that she wanted to wander upstairs and that she didn't want him or me to come along with her. This was fine with me, as I knew that it meant that she was moving more deeply into labor, and that's always a good thing. I could tell, though, that her husband's feelings were a little hurt (though he was too cool to express this). I reassured him that everything was fine. It wasn't long before she was feeling the urge to push. At this time, she was happy to sit on the bed and lean back into his arms. With each push, though, it seemed that she adjusted her position a little bit, so that little by little, he was less like an armchair and more like a mattress. Her baby was almost crowning when he suddenly gasped, "I'm having trouble breathing!" Her response was quick and final: "Stay there!" So he did. Their baby was soon born between all four of their legs, kicking them both. This was not the birth that he had imagined, but he couldn't have been more pleased. "This was probably as close as a man gets to feeling what it's like to give birth," he told us.

Moral of the story: it's good to be flexible.

Our mainstream culture outlines a rather limited role for new fathers: the distribution of cigars to relatives and friends. We have also seen a role that is frequently shown on the television birth shows—father-to-be as photographer. I have observed (and have also heard several fathers report) that being the photographer of the labor and birth often has the effect of separating him from the feelings and the reality of the event. Maybe it feels safer for him at the moment, but while he may be happy to have a few photos, he often feels a sense of loss from having separated himself from the immediacy of this important event in his life. At any rate, this is something to think about.

The camera is not the only electronic device that can distract the attention of a nervous father-to-be in the birth room. When a laboring woman has an epidural in place, the electronic fetal monitor has a way of becoming the central focus of the room with its hypnotic beeps, flashing lights, and the constant hum of its printer. I recommend that dads turn down the volume knob and perhaps cover the entire console with a towel.

Let's say that your partner decides to forego an epidural. Slow dancing or some time in the shower or a warm tub of water can be excellent ways of helping her get the right hormones flowing for labor to be effective. Labor has a real intensity to it, so don't be surprised at this. Don't forget to breathe as slowly and deeply as possible, as this will help your partner's ability to relax as well. Will you be able to keep her from having any doubts in her ability to keep going? You should know that even women who have already given birth before sometimes express this kind of uncertainty when they are almost fully dilated. This feeling almost always passes when pushing begins. Most likely the best way to help her get through this part is to be as close to her as she wants you to be and to be calm and steady for her. Pay close attention, and you will know what she needs.

WHAT'S THIS ABOUT A MONKEY?

Now we get to the last key concept: learning about your partner's monkey self. To explain this one more fully, I'm going to refer to an article that originally appeared in the *Missoula Independent* by Skylar Browning, a first-time father.[1]

> I heard about the monkey early on. It was during the first trimester of the pregnancy of our first child when our licensed midwife, Sandhano Danison, was telling a story about Mormon nurses in Idaho. The nurses had invited the godmother of the natural childbirth movement, Ina May Gaskin, to educate them on how to incorporate her values into their medical practices. One nurse couldn't wrap herself around the idea of not providing a woman in labor some sort of drug to relieve the pain. The nurse asked Ina May what she could possibly do to naturally comfort the woman. Ina May thought for a second and replied, "I would tell her to let her monkey do it." The Mormon nurses were much confused.
>
> "I'm not sure they knew what they were getting when they invited her to speak," said Sandhano, finishing the story with a laugh she shared with my wife.
>
> Suddenly I was lumped in with a group of Mormon nurses: I didn't get it. Whose monkey? What monkey? Nobody told me anything about a monkey. As I became accustomed to doing throughout the pregnancy, I asked what the heck was going on.
>
> Turns out, we all have a monkey. Whether we use it for giving birth or mountain biking, Ina May says if we

can short-circuit the mind during physical pursuit, we can let our inner primate do the work. "It's a short way of saying not to let your over-busy mind interfere with the ancient wisdom of your body," she writes in *Ina May's Guide to Childbirth*. "Monkeys don't think of technology as necessary to birth-giving; monkeys don't obsess about their bodies being inadequate . . . Monkeys don't do math about their dilation to speculate how long labor might take . . . Monkeys in labor get into the position that feels best, not the one they're told to assume . . ."

In other words, your monkey is a way to remember in the throes of labor that natural childbirth is not only possible, it's, well, natural.

My wife and I must have read more than 20 childbirth books between us (full disclosure: I only read two, but I heard a lot of "Hey, listen to this . . ."), we participated in a six-week birthing class, and Sandhano walked us through six months of prenatal visits, but as I wrestled with my inner uncertainties about natural childbirth at home, it was the idea that my wife would just let her monkey do it that resonated the most.

So it came to be that after 41 weeks of pregnancy and 20 hours of slowly progressing labor, my wife was crouched in an inflatable birthing tub—a really cool kiddy pool with some sort of *Finding Nemo*–like decorative patterning—situated smack-dab in the middle of our dining room. She began to shake uncontrollably at the onset of a contraction. Sandhano was catching a catnap in a corner and Charlotte Creekmore McCarvel, her apprentice, had crashed in the next room. I looked at my wife as the contraction ended and asked if things were okay.

"Wow, that was intense," she said for the first time in a day full of contractions.

I thought she was quivering from the water turning cold—after all, she'd been in there for some time—and suggested she get out. But as I grabbed the towel another contraction came, again preceded by her legs shaking in the water.

"Nicole, are you alright?" I asked, masking as best I could a slight panic.

Her face looked so focused. Concentrated. Not present. After 12 years as a couple, I'd never seen that expression before. I wrapped her in a towel and woke Sandhano. I had a feeling the monkey had arrived.

"What . . . if . . . something . . . goes . . . wrong?"

. . . I kept waiting for the monkey. Nicole's legs shook with electric rushes of adrenaline through her body, mighty currents of hormones and endorphins kicking in to help her through the process. Her eyes were closed, but I clasped her hands and with every contraction squeezed through it with her as Sandhano helped her follow rhythmic breathing patterns—Pah! Pah! Pah!

We moved from the birthing pool down to our bedroom, which had been set up earlier in the day. There was a fresh set of sheets atop a plastic cover, and under the plastic another set of clean sheets. The idea was that after the birth, the top sheets could be pulled off and Nicole, the baby and I could rest in a clean, ready-made bed. The sheets were just one of many steps we'd taken to prepare the house for this moment.

. . . On the bed, the contractions were still coming about five minutes apart, but they were becoming noticeably more intense. Nicole laid on her side, with me across from her. Sandhano occasionally checked the baby's heartbeat and Nicole's blood pressure, but for the most part it was just Nicole and I. Rather, I think it was mostly just Nicole—the glazed look she developed in the birthing tub had morphed even further into a deep, zoned stare. While she breathed and managed each contraction, I found myself watching her, befuddled and amazed. She was grunting. The sweat was so thick that her t-shirt (it had a picture of a smiling Buddha and read, "For good luck, rub my tummy") was soaked through, and heavy. I glanced at the clock and saw it was almost 4:00 AM; she was going on her 26th hour.

"I was in labor la-la-land," says Nicole. "Everything was really touch-oriented and all about my body. I could feel myself grabbing your hand and your bicep, and I could feel Sandhano rubbing my back. That was it."

For me this controlled chaos was actually comforting. For most of the day, and the previous night, we'd done very little out of the ordinary. After her initial contractions began, we went to bed. In the morning I cooked a small breakfast and we went for a walk through the neighborhood. In the afternoon, I conducted an interview for work. We listened to music and swung in the backyard hammock. The only thing that hinted Nicole was in labor was her occasional pause—she'd stop, grab her lower back, maybe grimace, and I'd ask, "Ya having one?" and she'd nod. Then we went back to a routine that seemed like a lazy Saturday. So when things actually began happening—when Nicole was pushing and Sandhano was coaching and Charlotte was preparing and I was trying to remain conscious (I'd been assured smelling salts were nearby, just in case)—the birth of our child finally felt real. And natural.

Knowing what to say to a woman in this stage of labor is like finding the right words to ask out a girl in junior high school—you know what you're supposed to say, and you practice all the time, but when the moment comes you inevitably shove a Teva directly in your mouth. I was doing all right throughout the 26 hours—lots of "I love you" and "You're amazing" and "You're doing great"—but at the end I slipped. When I inadvertently asked, "How are you feeling?" Nicole gave me a look of death. But when I played coach and said, "Make sure you're breathing," she combined that look with a pissed-off hiss: "I am breathing."

I remember that moment because it was one of the few times Nicole spoke during the whole ordeal. And because the next thing she said was, "This really hurts!"

That line—This really hurts—was the only time she ever hinted at the pain, at losing her edge. But instead of stopping or giving up, she flipped off her side and started to experiment with different birthing positions. She moved quickly and grunted hard when she pushed.

"When I was pushing at the end and it really hurt," she says, "I could imagine at that point why many women decide to take drugs. I wasn't thinking about monkeys or animals. I just wanted to push the baby out. I was doing whatever I could."

The only problem was the baby's heartbeat. It slowed in some of the positions Nicole tried, at one point dropping dangerously low. Charlotte hooked up an oxygen tank—the more oxygen Nicole received, the more for the baby. Sandhano became calmly assertive, directing Nicole into certain positions. Whether it was the monkey or something else, something had to happen soon for our baby to be born.

"I wasn't feeling any pain at all."

In our birthing class, I had scoffed at the idea of a birthing stool—basically a metal frame that simulates the sensation of sitting on a toilet—because it seemed so silly. It looked and sounded like the subject of some late-night infomercial where if you call now (!) you'll also get your own "Let your monkey do it" bumper sticker, all for the low, low price of $19.95. Little did I know that the birthing stool would become the secret weapon of Nicole's natural delivery.

With none of the positions working and the baby's heartbeat still struggling, Sandhano directed Nicole to the stool at the foot of the bed. Almost immediately, our baby was dropping like a pinball down the shoot, literally gaining momentum as gravity took hold. I was on the bed, behind Nicole, propping her up with all my might so her weight didn't press too hard against the metal frame. I stuck to repeating, "You're doing great."

In what felt like seconds, but was truly just minutes, I heard Sandhano say, "I need hands!" The next thing I saw, like a magic act, Nicole was holding our perfect baby daughter in her arms.

"As soon as I got onto the birthing stool, I knew I could do it. That position was the right position," she says. "It all came together there with you behind me holding me up and Sandhano and Charlotte positioned. I had all the support I needed."

Champagne never tasted so good at six in the morning. I popped the cork in our bedroom and poured glasses for everyone. Charlotte brought down sliced strawberries from our refrigerator, cheese and crackers and some "Labor-Aid" (Emergen-C, crushed calcium tablets, honey, lemon juice and water) to re-hydrate Nicole. Propped in our bed, Nicole was wide-awake, in perfect spirits and holding our daughter under new sheets. I was exhausted, mentally and physically drained and drinking Freixenet like a marathon runner drinks Dixie cups of water.

"I wasn't tired," Nicole says. "I wasn't feeling any pain at all."

She did admit there were times of doubt. Nicole never revealed them, never voiced her concern, but at points, she says, she wasn't sure she could finish the birth.

The longevity of the labor and the painful final moments are two points that can intimidate some women. Sandhano jokes about midwives being labeled masochists for challenging women to overcome such intense pain.

"But it's different from that," Sandhano says. "Birth is a mysterious process of opening up and letting go and finding out how much the human body and nature are capable of. I don't see it as pain like cutting your finger. I see it as an emotional experience."

It all goes back to the monkey.

"The whole time I was trying not to think about it and just to let go," says Nicole. "I wanted my body to take over because if it knew how to make this baby inside of me, it knew how to birth it."

... *Postscript: Annabella Rose Bradley Browning was born at 4:29 am on Saturday, July 16, weighing 6 lbs. and measuring 19.5 inches.*

THE FATHER'S ROLE AFTER THE BIRTH

No man who has seen his wife give birth positively, without intervention, can imagine denying her that opportunity next time.

—Adam Maclean, father of four

Even if your partner has the most perfect birth ever and your baby is born in perfect condition, your role as protector is not over. If her intention is to breast-feed, you can be of help by keeping the room as quiet as possible so that she and the baby can focus their attention on each other. Both will be in an especially sensitive state for the first hour or two following birth, and both will usually be alert and awake, making this the perfect time to touch each other and look into each other's eyes. Unless there is some compelling reason why either mother or baby needs medical attention, it is best for them to be in close contact with each other, preferably such that the fronts of their bodies are touching as much as possible. It's important to help your partner get comfortable in a way that allows her to relax all parts of her body; quite often it works well for mother to be leaning back and seated. It's best if there is only a light layer of clothing between them so mother and baby can feel each other's bodies. Your partner can benefit from your helping the rest of the family members understand why she and the baby need that tranquil initial hour or so with each other (and you, of course), without a great deal of distraction in the room.

I have met many young men who approach fatherhood assuming that they will be helping with food preparation and cleanup and other housework because they are already living this way. If you are not yet one of them, I hope that you will become part of the movement of your generation that is realizing that housework happens best when it is shared. Do you know how to cook healthy, delicious food? If so, you already know how much this will help. If not, it's never too late to learn!

If you are a father-to-be and, after reading this chapter, the prospect of being present during labor and the birth of your child seems daunting, I suggest that you watch the wonderful film *March of the Penguins*. Those emperor penguins really know how to "father," and if you haven't already seen this amazing documentary, I'm sure that you will feel inspired after watching it.

NOTE
1. Reprinted with the permission of the author.

Keri at The Farm

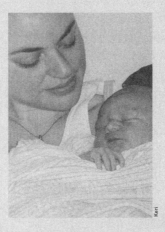

Keri

When I first discovered I was expecting, I immediately stepped up the research I had begun months before. A friend who knows me well suggested that I view a documentary video called *The Business of Being Born*, made by former talk show host Ricki Lake and Abby Epstein. The video introduced me to the merits of home birth and showed me what hospital birthing had become over the last several decades. The statistics were jarring, and the view of what birth could be was enlightening.

Watching *The Business of Being Born* was a jumping-off place for me, one that led me to Ina May's books. The first one I read was her *Ina May's Guide to Childbirth*. This sounds like a cliché, but it changed my life by changing my views on childbirth, pregnancy, breast-feeding, my own body, my womanhood, and certainly how I wanted to bring my baby into this world. It turned me into a sponge for information and eventually into an activist in my own right. It made me realize that having a baby is not just about the healthy child at the end of the journey, as so many claim. Pregnancy and childbirth is a pivotal point in a woman's life. The positive or negative feelings a woman experiences during this event can determine the course of the birth, and these feelings can, and often will, alter her forever. Birth is a rite of passage not to be taken lightly and not to be molested. This experience can be incredibly traumatizing to a woman, or it can be spiritual and transformative.

I interviewed four Certified Nurse Midwives, or CNMs, from three different ob-gyn practices. I knew I wanted the closest thing to The Farm experience as I could get. I spent at least fifteen minutes explaining my ideal birth to these midwives and I was amazed at the response. I immediately felt them giving me the "Oh, you are one of those!" looks. They handed me what seemed like hundreds of pamphlets on genetic testing, scary risk factors, what to avoid while pregnant. I felt like I was being treated like someone with an illness rather than someone who was about to experience a completely normal physiological event.

For each midwife I asked a standard question: "If I come into the hospital in labor, and for some reason the labor stops or slows, what will be your first step?" The answer was the same for all four: "We will start you on a Pitocin drip." They didn't offer the option of sending me home, or stimulating my nipples with a breast pump to encourage the release of oxytocin, which could start contractions. They didn't say they would suggest a walk to get things moving. After listening to me talk for fifteen minutes about my desire for a completely natural birth with no interventions or drugs the only suggestion they could offer me was an IV drip of a synthetic oxytocin called Pitocin, a drug that is known to make contractions stronger than they would normally be and harder to handle without pain relief.

Then, they gave me a form to sign. At eight weeks pregnant I was still at least thirty-two weeks from birth. I was a rookie, and I knew little about pregnancy. The form stated that by signing it, I would be giving all rights to the doctor on call to make whatever decisions he felt were warranted at the time. He need not ask me in the moment. They were asking me to trust someone I had never met to make decisions about my physical health and well-being (and that of my child) without consulting me. What was more, I had to sign it before leaving that day if I wanted to make another prenatal appointment. I refused and asked for my records.

I began wondering if it was even possible to give birth in my state (or many places in the US) in the way that I had come to see as ideal. If I asked for and sought out a natural birth, how good were the odds that I would have one? Would a birth plan be honored or even considered? Would it be too easy for me to "risk out" and end up caught up in the wave of interventions in which my friends had found themselves?

After considering all of this carefully, I made arrangements to give birth at The Farm. When I arrived there, I immediately fell in love with both the Farm and Pamela, who would be our midwife, and knew that this was exactly what I wanted. Only a week before I had been examined by a midwife in an ob-gyn practice in my hometown. She asked me if I had been sexually molested because of my reaction to her touch. During that same type of exam with Pamela, she was able to tell me how wide the spread of the inside of my pelvis was with her hand without me even knowing she had been that far inside me. This woman had skill. She also had tenderness. There was a calm, welcoming warmth in everything about her and our first prenatal visit. She knew not only how to birth babies, but also how to treat women. When I read The Farm contract I was expecting a little bit of what I had experienced at home, some sort of "locking in," but there was nothing—just straight forward, easy to understand, we-work-for-you kind of stuff. I signed.

I'd like it if we could put something here like "Before I knew it, it was time to prepare for my birth and head to the Farm," because otherwise it sounds like I lived on The Farm or had Pamela for all of my prenatal care. Instead, once I arrived on The Farm, every week I went to a clinic for my prenatal checkups. However, Pamela and I spent a little time with each other every day so she always knew how

I was feeling and closely monitored my progress, diet, and emotional state. The weekend of May 15th brought my estimated due date, and with it, loads of symptoms. I had been contracting for weeks but on that Saturday, they became pretty intense. I started having some loose bowel movements and menstrual-type cramps. Both, I was told, were signs of labor. On a walk that morning I even had multiple orgasms as I contracted! I had heard this was possible but didn't think for a second I could be one of the few lucky ones who experience it.

All day, I had a funny high which left me feeling really out-of-body. Pamela attributed this to surges in my levels of oxytocin and estrogen. She checked me and found that I was nearly completely effaced (thinned out) and about a centimeter dilated. She said the baby's head was very low.

But that day ended and no labor. Life went on and another weekly prenatal came and went. We hoped it would be my last, and indeed it was. I found out that Deborah Flowers, another Farm midwife, was interested in attending my labor. She had come to my last two prenatal visits. I felt so honored to have two amazing women who were quite legendary planning to help bring my baby into the world.

Friday, May 21st came and went with the return of that high being the only symptom I felt. I was talking to my mother on the computer and felt very out-of-body and happy.

The next morning, I awoke to what I imagined was a little bloody show. By lunchtime, I was contracting with pressure. I walked to The Farm's store to have lunch and talked to Louise and Donna (the women who work there) for about an hour. I paid a quick hello to Deborah, who was outside under the dome having lunch with some others. It was then that I felt a contraction that made me feel the need to steady myself. By this time I suspected labor might be starting and headed home to my cabin.

I spent some time over at Pamela's house with Pamela and some of her friends who were visiting. All the time my contractions were becoming more regular and more intense. I was excited but didn't want to get my hopes up in case it was another false alarm like the weekend before. I sent a text message to my mother and mentioned that I thought I "might" be in labor. Soon after, it appeared that this was in fact the real thing and I could deny it no longer. I went to the bathroom and there was a little more blood. Tamami, one of the women who was visiting Pamela, massaged my back through a couple of contractions. I began to feel like I wanted to put things in order and decided to go to my cabin.

Another friend of Pamela's stayed with me during my early labor. I didn't know her well and found that I began to get self-conscious about the moaning and vocalizing I was doing to manage my contractions, so I went into the bathroom and closed the door with each one. Soon, I wasn't leaving the bathroom at all. Instead I paced back and forth rubbing my abdomen between the contractions and leaned on the bathroom counter when they peaked, looking myself in the mirror and moaning. I realized that soon my moaning turned into a melodic hum. I recognized it as the song the black soldiers hummed between prayers and thoughts the night before they went into battle in the film *Glory*. I thought that was interesting, because it was completely unplanned and seemingly instinctual. Before I went into labor I had no idea what I would do to manage pain or discomfort. I hadn't planned any methods or taken any classes. Everything I was doing was what felt right at the time, but I would never have expected what I did. Fortunately, it was incredibly effective and I was able to manage the pain very well.

Pamela came in and said it seemed that I was progressing quickly and she wanted to set up the birthing tub. Her words didn't really sink in until later. At this time, I was under the assumption that this was the beginning of a very long process. This being my first baby, I had heard that women often labored for twenty-four hours or longer, so I believed I had a long stretch ahead of me. She wanted to check me. She said I was completely effaced and about two centimeters dilated. She went back home to gather the materials to set up the tub.

About fifteen to twenty minutes later the tub was up and being filled. I was pacing harder and faster, moaning louder and more often. I didn't really want or need any assistance from anyone at this time and preferred to stay in the bathroom by myself. Conversation was difficult and threw me off my focus. I was somewhat aware of Pamela coming in and out of the cabin and preparing her equipment, but my focus was on my breathing and my humming. Pamela mentioned she had "no desire to leave me" but wanted to start setting up for the birth and needed to go back to her house to gather more of her supplies. She said she would be right back to check me again. When she did, she found I was four centimeters dilated.

It was a humid day and I felt that the bathroom, with its window air conditioning unit, was really the only place I was comfortable. I also felt a bit on display when I left this sanctuary, which doesn't sit well with me when I am feeling vulnerable. So I went back in and continued to pace the bathroom, rubbing my abdomen in big circular motions as I walked. It seemed the only place I could concentrate on the contractions.

It got to the point where time was starting to not make much sense to me. Pamela checked me again after what seemed a very short period of time. I was too wrapped up in managing my breathing and concentrating on the contractions. She discovered I was now at eight centimeters.

I had been looking forward to using the birthing tub. I had heard that it was a great way to relax and reduce the discomfort of the contractions. Pamela had explained that she didn't like to have her birthing mothers use the tub until they were at least six centimeters, as it could sometimes slow down labor. Now that I was past that point, she gave me the go-ahead and I climbed into the hot water. It definitely did slow the contractions and reduce their intensity but I couldn't stay in long. Within only a few minutes the water had me out of breath and completely overheated. I climbed out and headed for the bathroom again to cool off and regain my lost control.

During the next several moments, I heard Pamela on the phone telling the other two midwives, Stacie and Deborah, that if they wanted to be there for the birth, they needed to hurry over now. It wasn't until that moment that I realized that Pamela was implying that this would be a fast labor. It wouldn't be long before my little one would be joining us.

By the time they arrived, I was nine centimeters dilated. At this point, I felt the urge to push. I was surprised to find that the sensation was not what I expected. It felt like if I didn't hold my butt cheeks tightly together I could lose my stuff—like I would take a crap right there on the bed. The contractions had gone from really intense to nearly overwhelming. I know now that this was transition. I have to admit, at this point, I felt like I was drowning. Panic hit me for the first time.

Deborah was on one side of me and Stacie was on the other while Pamela remained between my legs. I felt too tired at this point to walk anymore and I couldn't concentrate on the contractions without help, but I hated lying down. I actually felt the irrational urge to run from the feelings I was having, as if I could escape my own body.

Sensing this, Deborah got my attention and said, "Look at me and slow your breathing, Keri . . . Slooooooooow in . . . Slooooooow out," and as I breathed with her she praised me. She coached me through a few breaths, and then the contraction had passed and I was calm again. Pamela checked me again and triumphantly announced that I was at ten centimeters and I could push whenever I was ready.

At that moment, I realized, really realized, that I was having a baby. Just like all the fictional and documentary videos I had seen with women grunting and panting, legs spread, people surrounding them, I was about to have a baby.

The contractions now felt just like an overwhelming need to have a bowel movement. Why did I not know that? I thought of all the women who talked of their fears of pooping on the delivery table. Now consider this: there is no person I know who has bigger bathroom phobias and hang-ups than I do, but at that moment, I said to myself, "OK, so if you shit on the bed in front of everyone, then you shit on the bed in front of everyone. So what? You need to have this baby and there is only one way to do it."

So with each contraction, I gripped the hand of Deborah on my right and the hand of Stacie on my left, pulled myself upright and bore down with everything I had, like I was taking a massive poop right there in front of poor Pamela.

This went on for what seemed like forever, and I could feel the baby moving down. I could feel it move back ever so slightly inside me for every little bit of progress forward. I felt myself stretching. I visualized a film I had seen just days before when the baby's head was crowning and then came out with only the body left to be born and I tried to visualize my own baby doing the same and focus on working toward that.

I screamed, I roared like a lion. I felt so dramatic but it seemed to work for me. I never thought I would be one to yell but here I was doing it. I apologized for my drama. The women all laughed and said it was fine. I didn't need to apologize for anything. They said I was doing a wonderful job and they could feel and see the head of the baby getting closer. I pushed and pushed. I felt overheated again and asked for something to cool me down. Someone put a cold, wet washcloth on my forehead and they gave me water. I wondered if I could do this any longer.

The pushing helped with the contractions. If I didn't push hard they were more uncomfortable. I began to wonder if I would tear and thought I should just do it. So what if I tore? Women had before and survived, and so would I. But I confess, I was a tiny bit afraid of that. Up to this point of my pregnancy I had had absolutely no fear of labor and delivery, which I thought was pretty amazing. But here I was wondering, "Will I survive this? Will it ever end?" The women reassured me that there was nothing to be afraid of, I was doing great and the baby was coming. "You are having your baby!" they told me. And I was. They asked me if I wanted to see my progress in a hand mirror. I said "No! Just get this baby out of me!" (I did say "kid" but in retrospect that sounds awful.)

The last few pushes I felt the burn I had been warned about. It was what scared me the most. It didn't last long but it was intense and I pushed with everything I had despite it just to bring it to an end. Then, just like that, I felt the head come out. I paused for what seemed only a second to catch my breath as they congratulated me and some fussing was being done, probably to clear the baby's airway, and I said to myself, "OK, no sense in prolonging this any further." With the next contraction I spit the rest of my child out. That is exactly what it felt like, and the relief was instant and complete.

In a flurry of activity, they were wrapping him in a blanket and putting him on my belly. All I could say was "I had a baby!" over and over. Then, before I knew he was a boy, I said, "He is so handsome!" Feeling silly for saying this about a potential baby girl, I took a look down below and confirmed my baby was indeed a little boy.

The next few minutes were a blur as I heard Pamela say that the cord was pulsing and she was preparing to cut it once it stopped. I watched her clamp and cut it. They began talking about the placenta and how easy it would be to deliver because there were no bones in it and I was thinking, "Oh right, there is one last thing . . . well, let's do this and be done with it all!" I didn't even wait for a contraction. I just pushed and out it came. In that moment I rejoiced. My pregnancy, labor, and delivery were complete.

He was eight pounds and fourteen ounces, and twenty-one inches long. I had delivered him in five and a half hours and pushed for forty-five minutes. This was impressive, they said, for a first baby and for a baby so large. Pamela described me as an efficient birther. She also mentioned how neat I was. The baby came out relatively clean with not much blood or any vernix.

I was a mommy! My love for this little guy was something I could never have fathomed. I realized that all the inconvenience of driving down to Tennessee, eighteen hours from home, defending my reasons for doing so over and over and over to doubting friends and family ... was all worth it. I never had so much as an IV. I was not exposed to Pitocin, an epidural, dilation drugs like Cervidil, or drugs used off label for birth like Cytotec. There were no hospital gowns, fetal monitors, hospital beds, or policies, no shift changes or strangers. My baby was born in the cabin I had lived in for a month, on the bed I slept in every night, among women I had grown to love and trust. I was free to labor in whatever way felt comfortable to me. I had made the journey from a girl to a woman, and from a woman to a mother. I had done it all trusting that my body was designed to birth my baby with little fear. And I felt like I could do anything.

—Keri

CHAPTER 8

My Vision for the Future

Everything has to be in balance . . . We do not know how to listen and
hear the people who have good things to tell us. All of these things have
to be kept in the balance—the listening and the speaking, the male and the
female, the clan mother and the chiefs, and all of the people in between . . .
The women within our own society have a special place of honor. We
have the ability to bring forth life to this earth.

—Audrey Shenandoah, Clan Mother of the Onondaga Nation

You can always count on Americans to do the right thing—after
they've tried everything else.

—Winston Churchill

WOMAN-CENTERED MATERNITY CARE IS A HUMAN RIGHT

Having the chance to travel to many countries has allowed me to
meet midwives, physicians, and (more recently) doulas who work
within maternity care systems that are very different from what we
have in the US. Every country I have visited (except Brazil) has a
reverse ratio of midwives to physicians compared to what we have
here, meaning that their midwives far outnumber physicians
involved in maternity care. People who live in countries where there
has always been a midwifery profession consider it a rational health
care policy for midwives to be the providers of maternity care for
approximately 70 percent of pregnant women. By contrast, people
in the US tend to think that every pregnancy requires an obstetrician and that midwives are some kind of more recent fad. The ratio
of midwives to obstetricians in the UK, for instance, is thirty-five

midwives to one obstetrician, according to the Royal College of Midwives and the Royal College of Obstetricians and Gynaecologists. About 35,000 midwives are available to care for about 650,000 births in the UK. In the US, we have about 8,000 midwives to care for more than 4.1 million births, so relatively few US women have the option of having a midwife, even if they want one and even if there is no other maternity care professional in their area. I think that at least 100,000 midwives and a total of 4,000 to 5,000 physicians would be a more reasonable demographic for maternity care providers for the future in the US. We should shift away from continuing to educate maternity nurses, and instead use our resources to educate more midwives (some of whom, of course, would be maternity nurses with additional midwifery training).

At present, it is hard to find out who in the Department of Health and Human Services (HHS) approves the funding for the training of health professionals and makes the decisions as to which professionals receive the most funding for training. Marsden Wagner attempted to get answers to this question from HHS officials, with little success, despite hours on the phone.[1] There should be far more transparency surrounding this process. It's a pretty safe assumption that ACOG currently has the greatest influence among professional groups on HHS maternity care policy, since its residents now receive the lion's share of federal funds and subsidies. This also must change in favor of training more midwives. The national Medicaid program that currently pays hospitals to train residents should shift these payments to train midwives. Medicaid should also fund efficient distance education programs such as the Frontier School of Midwifery and Family Nursing's CNEP program, which produces more midwives and nurse practitioners each year than any other program in the country. Nurses who have graduated as registered nurses, who plan to work in obstetrics wards but who have not really learned the skills of helping women to labor effectively, should go through doula training and get this kind of certification as well.

With such changes in place, it would be possible for practice groups to develop that would include two obstetricians, six midwives, and six doulas. Such teams would be able to produce better outcomes with fewer C-sections. Furthermore, state laws and regulations need to change so that midwives can practice independently without having to report to doctors. All states should license both nurse-midwives and direct-entry midwives.

Here's an important statistic: 49 percent of US counties have no obstetrician at all, because they are located in rural areas. The ACOG interprets this fact to mean that fifty-two thousand obstetricians aren't enough, even though very few are willing or able to live and work in small towns and rural areas across the country. High malpractice premiums for obstetricians in some states call for higher-volume practices than some areas can offer. Twenty-five percent of the US population—about 77 million people—live in rural areas, but only 10 percent of doctors practice there and only a few of these—mostly family physicians—provide maternity care. A 2010 bulletin from the American Association of Retired Persons featured an article about a family doctor who works in a town of 1,200 in northern Montana. The only doctor within a radius of at least forty miles in all directions, he works alone and is constantly on call, without backup. It is difficult for him to arrange for a vacation. Because he is not set up to provide prenatal care or to attend births, every pregnant woman in his area has to drive or be driven 120 miles away for maternity care. Not surprisingly, some babies are born in cars, without any qualified person attending, en route.[2]

Just over the border in Canada, the towns are just as small and the cities just as far apart, but family physicians and midwives there take part in a collaborative effort to extend care to rural populations. My dream is to see a similar kind of collaboration take place in the US. I know that it is possible, because a few family doctors and midwives are already working together in this way. However, for these kinds of partnerships to happen in the areas where they are needed, we must have stronger incentives to increase both the number of family physicians and midwives of all kinds (certified nurse-midwives [CNMs], certified professional midwives [CPMs], and certified midwives [CMs]) willing to work together in areas that lack maternity services. It is important for us to remove all obstacles preventing family physicians and midwives from filling the gaps that now exist in nearly half of US counties. At this writing, twenty-five more states need to pass laws that expand access to CPMs, thus joining the twenty-five states that now recognize this category of midwives (which includes yours truly). I recommend that women's groups join the Big Push for Midwives campaign that is actively working to expand out-of-hospital maternity care options in the US. See the Resources section for ways to link up with this campaign and other consumer efforts that work for the same or similar goals. Don't take no for an answer! Remember the suffragists and their struggles, which still benefit us today.

REVISE MEDICAL EDUCATION

The best obstetricians are those who had midwives as teachers of normal birth, who gave them a good grounding in the normal process of labor and birth before they entered the part of their training pertaining to obstetrical pathology. Such training instills respect for midwives and recognition of the mind-body connection that is so necessary a part of the knowledge base for any medical professional in maternity care. Sphincter law should be part of the curriculum, as well as a thorough knowledge of the emotional states that are associated with the ecstatic hormones of birth. Every obstetrician in training should have an opportunity to witness (at least on video) an ecstatic birth. Medical and midwifery students should have a chance to watch nature in action by viewing videos of large mammals giving birth without human interference. With midwives as teachers, doctors in training would be able to learn some of the ancient midwifery techniques that would help to lower C-section rates if they were applied across the country. These ingenious techniques include the all-fours (or Gaskin) maneuver to solve the complication of shoulder dystocia (stuck shoulders), which I learned from indigenous Guatemalan midwives, who told me they had learned it from God; the use of a long shawl called a rebozo to change a baby's position; massage techniques; and the use of upright postures and movement during labor. Techniques of manual assessment of pelvic dimensions, fetal size, and breech delivery need to be revived and taught. Medical schools in other countries manage to teach breech skills to both medical and midwifery students with the use of mannequins and models; we can do the same. Physicians in training need to learn how to perform vaginal examinations that don't make the woman feel violated. All medical professionals should be exposed to at least the broad outlines of medical and midwifery history as part of their training. Finally, every future obstetrician ought to dress at least two newborn babies early in their training so they can become more familiar with how to handle them with tenderness and so they can have the confidence that they won't be hurting them.

I am indebted to Drs. Charles Mahan and Marsden Wagner for having already articulated several of these proposals; Dr. Mahan did so in his foreword to Nicette Jukelevics's excellent book *Understanding the Dangers of Cesarean Birth*, and Dr. Wagner did so in his essential *Born in the USA: How a Broken Maternity Care System Must be Fixed to Put Women and Children First*.[3]

ESTABLISH MATERNITY CARE STANDARDS

We need medical practice standards at both the federal and the state level that would address C-sections performed without medical justification, and assure more mother-friendly births and fewer medical interventions during labor. Brazil has already begun to establish such measures, such that hospitals receive less payment from government insurance if their C-section rates exceed the standards. It is important to remember, as Dr. Mahan has pointed out, that "medicine is the only major industry in the US where reimbursement for services is not linked to adherence to a set of scientific evidence-based standards."[4] For a thorough summary of what maternity care standards I am talking about, please see the Mother-Friendly Childbirth Initiative in the appendix.

Furthermore, insurance payers, whether public or private, should have to pay according to the performance and outcome standards mentioned above. If the payers refuse to pay for certain services (vaginal births after cesarean, for instance), people who care should meet with their state government insurance commissioners and pressure them to do the right thing. Lobby your local legislator to put pressure on your state Medicaid program directors to raise the rates for birth services. Dr. Mahan suggests that VBAC reimbursement should be raised to $2,000; that a vaginal birth reimbursement be $1,800; and that C-section reimbursement be placed at $1,000.

PHYSICIANS SHOULD BE SALARIED AND NOT PAID BY THE NUMBER OF BIRTHS THEY TAKE ON

The rationale for this recommendation is that it would prevent obstetricians from taking on more births than they should, along with the gynecological surgeries they are additionally responsible for. The nearly unchecked freedom many now enjoy means that many women's labors are accelerated, or they are pressured to consent to a C-section that is really unnecessary, so the physician can go home for family time or a good night's sleep. It's a national disgrace that the CDC's statistics now show that more C-sections are performed between 5:00 and 6:00 PM than at any other time of day.

BIRTH CENTERS ARE NEEDED IN ALL PARTS OF THE US

The US National Birth Center Study, published in the *New England Journal of Medicine* in 1989, looked at eighty-four freestanding birth centers staffed by nurse-midwives and the total of 11,814 births that they attended. There were no maternal deaths at all in the study. The rate of perinatal deaths (1.3 per 1,000 live births) was comparable to the rates among low-risk hospital births, and only 16 percent of the birth center births were transferred to hospitals because of complications. Birth centers differ from hospitals in that women giving birth in a birth center can expect their midwives to stay with them throughout the course of labor, whereas in a hospital they can be on the point of giving birth when they have to say good-bye to the midwife who had been with them for hours because of a shift change. Women using birth centers have far fewer induced births (since midwives are less likely to push for induction) and fewer C-sections. Their babies are less likely to be taken away from them just following birth, because habitual hospital routines such as unnecessary separation of mother and baby have not been instituted at birth centers.

Japan has long had neighborhood birth houses as one of the choices of birth place that women have available to them, and has birth outcomes that are superior to those in the US. Such birth houses were part of Japanese birth culture throughout most of the twentieth century, and there is a growing network in Japan that is calling for more of them to be established. Germany, a country in which there were almost no birth centers previous to 1990, has seen a tremendous growth in the number of them. By 2000, there were more than seventy. Any country the size of our own ought to have tens of thousands of birth centers for those healthy women who would like a middle-ground alternative to a hospital or home birth. Such birth centers would be staffed by CNMs, CPMs, or CMs, who would be backed up by physicians with obstetrical privileges at a nearby hospital. Despite the good results of birth centers and their popularity with women, extremely high malpractice insurance rates and physician opposition have forced many independent birth centers to close their doors. Birth centers need protection from the economic and legislative advantages currently enjoyed by hospital corporations, which don't appreciate the competition they pose to area hospitals, and obstetricians, who don't want midwives competing with them. In the early eighties, there were 400 freestanding birth centers. In 2005, there were only 160.

EVERY MATERNAL DEATH MUST BE COUNTED AND REVIEWED

It is simply unacceptable that a US woman giving birth today has a greater chance of dying than her mother did. If we want to reverse this trend (and this is possible), there is an essential step that we must take in order to know the causes of our sharply rising maternal death rate and attempt to address them. *We have to set up—for the first time—a national system that makes it possible to identify and count every maternal death.* Unless every death is identified and reviewed, it is not possible to know the causes of all deaths or their actual frequency, and then to work to prevent them. Just as every airplane crash must be thoroughly investigated (it would be unthinkable not to), every possible maternal death deserves a high level of attention.

At present, we have nothing more than an honor system of maternal death reporting, which produces such inaccurate numbers that the CDC reported in 1998 that the actual number could be three times greater than the number officially reported each year.[5] Almost nothing has been done since then to remedy the problem of a maternal death rate that is "grossly understated," in the words of one CDC epidemiologist.[6] Until we in the US organize to create such a system, we must realize that a significant number of women who die from pregnancy-related causes don't even enjoy the right to be a statistic, because their deaths go uncounted.

Other countries, with less wealth than ours, have created systems that achieve accurate counts of maternal deaths, so no one can argue that this task is impossible. It can be done. If it is not done, our country cannot arrive at definitive answers as to the reasons for maternal deaths, at least half of which are preventable, according to the CDC. So we must ask ourselves: do we Americans value our women enough to set up the necessary system for identifying and counting maternal deaths? Who would argue that we shouldn't, especially now that we know that our death rate is rising rather sharply?

We can turn to the UK for a good model. Every three years the Royal College of Obstetricians and Gynaecologists publishes a 300-page book entitled *Saving Mothers' Lives*. Anyone in Wales, Scotland, England, and Northern Ireland, the four countries of the United Kingdom, can walk into a bookstore and buy the book, or simply download it for free from the Internet. It is a sort of report card on the results of the combined maternity services of the UK. As the public outreach component of the UK's respected Confidential Enquiry into Maternal and Child Health (CEMACH), each edition of *Saving Mothers' Lives* is based on data drawn from every maternal death by causes stemming from pregnancy or birth during the preceding three years of available data. Each of the main causes of maternal deaths— hypertension, thromboembolism, hemorrhage, amniotic fluid embolism, infection, and anesthesia complications—gets its own chapter, and includes at least one vignette of a case of such a death.[7]

The CEMACH system is considered the gold standard in the world for professional self-audit in maternity care. Because its purpose is to get at the truth, names and places are kept confidential so that results of the inquiries can't be used in malpractice lawsuits. *Saving Mothers' Lives* not only provides detailed, accurate numbers for each category of death, but also makes recommendations about what steps should be taken to ensure that the number of deaths will be reduced in the next three-year period. And UK taxpayers are getting their money's worth, because the effect of the Confidential Enquiry is indisputably lifesaving. Its 2004 report could boast a twelve-fold improvement in maternal deaths compared with fifty years earlier and no report yet has had to record a significant rise in the death rate over the previous triennium. *The equivalent publication in the US is a mere two pages buried in the National Center for Health Statistics's yearly report, which is far from easy for the public to access.*[8] We can and must do better than that.

The doctors and public health authorities who created the UK's system of maternal death reporting began with a goal of achieving total assessment of deaths so that health professionals might learn from errors that may have contributed to some of the deaths. As doctors themselves, they understood that the system would have to be both confidential and mandatory. They also recognized that it doesn't make public health sense for hospitals to investigate themselves—that is, to conduct secretive in-house reviews of maternal deaths with only partial information about what happened. They wanted a way in which a mistake made in one or two institutions could provide lessons for the rest of a country's maternity wards.

I have spoken with CDC experts on maternal mortality, epidemiologists, and physicians, and they all agree that impartial review of every maternal death is necessary and cannot occur unless we have a revolution in our thinking and action in the area of preventing maternal deaths. If the CDC and the National Center for Health Statistics could by themselves fix what is wrong with our data gathering, review, and analysis relevant to making motherhood safer, they would already have done so, because they have been aware of the underreporting of maternal deaths since at least the midnineties. A lot of people who do not currently work for either agency are going to have to care about establishing a US system that works as well as the UK's CEMACH system. We need to educate ourselves and as many others as possible and organize to make this happen.

The focus of the US's current method of collecting and reviewing information about maternal deaths must shift from protection of the hospital and its staff from malpractice lawsuit to prevention of medical error. There is no penalty for inaccurate reporting, so the large degree of underreporting documented by the CDC should not surprise us. It should be clear that we are going to have to create incentives to report comprehensively and accurately, and fines for misreporting will most likely be necessary.

A LIST OF STEPS TO REDUCE THE US MATERNAL DEATH RATE

A "To Do" list for the revolutionary change required to gather accurate maternal death information and then to use it to prevent those deaths, where possible, follows. Once we have accomplished these steps, the answers for further progress will hopefully emerge.

◆ *Make every one of the fifty states use the US Standard Death Certificate, so that for the first time in our history, we would have consistency in how data on maternal death is gathered.*
    At this writing, nineteen states have death certificates that don't ask the same questions as those in the US Standard Death Certificate. This means that many maternal deaths are not recorded as such. This makes no sense.

◆ *Create effective penalties for misreporting, misclassifying, or falsifying information on death certificates.*
    The US has functioned too long with its honor system for us to expect that habits can change in this area unless there are powerful incentives to do so. This step will be necessary to create a new culture of honesty and a system-wide devotion to accuracy. Periodic, unannounced audits will be necessary.

◆ *Create and require training programs for doctors and anyone else authorized to fill in a death certificate in maternity hospitals.*
    Special training is necessary for filling out death certificates, according to the CDC. In its recent publication *Strategies to*

Reduce Pregnancy-Related Deaths, the CDC reports that "[p]hysicians receive minimal training in how to correctly complete death certificates. The cause of death on many certificates does not adequately reflect the events leading to the death, as evidenced by the under-assessment of pregnancy-related deaths when case identification is based solely on death certificate data."[9] This information is too important to be trusted to overtired residents who are leery of phoning a senior doctor in the middle of the night. And, in the interest of data consistency, the same standards and training must be followed nationwide.

♦ *Pass legislation at the national level to provide confidentiality to state maternal mortality review committees.*
Confidentiality is the cornerstone of CEMACH. Without it, the UK system would not be able to obtain complete medical and social records for each deceased mother and subject them to case review external to the hospital in question.

♦ *Require that insurance companies pay for an autopsy following the death of a woman of childbearing age in every case where the family agrees to the autopsy, to help contribute to research that will prevent deaths in the future. Countries with national health care systems do this as a matter of course, since it contributes to preventing more deaths (their main priority).*
Without autopsy, studies show that the wrong diagnosis for maternal death occurs between 25 and 40 percent of the time. Without precise diagnosis, ignorance and myth prevail, and lessons that should be learned cannot be learned. Autopsies, although they are necessary for medical research, medical education, and quality control, do not generate profit for hospitals.[10] Because insurance doesn't usually pay for such autopsies, the current autopsy rates for hospital deaths at nonteaching hospitals is estimated to be less than 9 percent, whereas in 1960, autopsy followed death in at least half of cases.[11]

- *Encourage the American Congress of Obstetricians and Gynecologists to emulate the example of its UK counterpart, the Royal College of Obstetricians and Gynaecologists, by periodically publishing a detailed and informative book as part of its effort to identify, review, study, and learn from maternal deaths in the US.*

POSTPARTUM HOME VISITS MUST BE RECOGNIZED AS A NECESSITY

When I began documenting US women's maternal deaths in the late nineties, I had not expected to find out that some women die from lack of postpartum care. A midwife friend of mine from New York mailed me a news article about a young Army specialist, Tameka McFarquhar, who had no family members nearby to help her when she was released from Samaritan Medical Center in Watertown, New York, a day after giving birth to her first child on December 14, 2004. A single mother, the Jamaican-born twenty-two-year-old had been transferred Stateside from Army duty in South Korea after becoming pregnant with her daughter, Danasia Elizabeth.

She spoke to her mother in Jamaica on the night of December 19 and told her that she had a headache. Worried about her, her mother advised her to drink some milk and keep herself warm.

That phone call was the last time that any family member or friend heard McFarquhar's voice. No one could get her to answer her phone or her apartment door. A concerned friend notified the Watertown police, who found no probable cause to break into the apartment. Finally, on Christmas morning, McFarquhar's friend again contacted the police, who this time went to McFarquhar's apartment, only to find a horrifying scene. McFarquhar had bled to death several days earlier, and baby Danasia had died of dehydration and starvation.[12]

Tameka McFarquhar had medical insurance. What is noteworthy is that her death certainly could have been prevented if she had had a postpartum home visit by a trained professional such as a midwife or specially trained nurse, the kind of visit that most countries that also have early hospital discharge after birth routinely provide for new mothers. Such visits are meant to catch problems which may not be detected at hospital discharge but develop during the first week or ten days following birth. Phone calls are not sufficient, since what is needed is a trained person who examines mother and baby. Retained material in the uterus will make the uterus especially tender, and it will create an odor that is unmistakable (but which the mother herself can't be expected to diagnose).

Postpartum home visits are important for many reasons: to detect early signs of postpartum depression, which sometimes escalates to postpartum psychosis; to help with breast-feeding problems; to answer questions the new parents might have about early infant care; to check for an infection that might not have been apparent on discharge; and to make sure that mothers, especially those who have had C-sections, are not showing signs of deep vein thrombosis. Several quilt blocks have been made for the Safe Motherhood Quilt Project for mothers who died of pulmonary embolism. Lara Nuerge Schultz, for instance, was limping three weeks after her C-section, a fact that her mother-in-law, a registered nurse, noticed. She tried but failed to persuade her daughter-in-law to seek immediate medical attention and pressured her son to take Lara to the hospital for care. Instead, Lara, unaware of the danger she was in, went on a long car trip to visit her ageing grandfather and died on the way home. Her story and several others have persuaded me that US women, especially those who have had C-sections, aren't being informed about the symptoms of pulmonary embolism (a painful swelling that may be hot to touch and usually develops in a leg).[13]

We cannot expect new mothers or family members to diagnose their own postpartum complications. With almost half of births being to single mothers, it is even more ridiculous to expect single mothers to be able to diagnose any complications by themselves. Home birth midwives provide postpartum visits during the days following birth as part of their routine services. However, it is relatively unusual for US hospital maternity services to include even one postpartum home visit. Instead, most services provide only for a six-week checkup at the doctor's office. Clearly, a six-week visit would not have been enough to save the lives of Tameka McFarquhar and her daughter. My vision for the future is that when single-payer health care comes about in the US, postpartum home visits are included as part of the needed services for new mothers.

WE MUST GIVE MORE CONSIDERATION TO A CATEGORY OF MOTHERS WHO NEED IT

In 2010, a new television series was launched in the US entitled *I Didn't Know I was Pregnant*. The series is teaching people that intelligent women can be pregnant and go into labor without realizing that they have a baby coming. In some cases, these surprise births occur in women who have already given birth before but who fail, for a variety of reasons, to recognize the symptoms of pregnancy or labor. However, when that same phenomenon happens in the case of a teenager and complications arise (for example, her baby doesn't spontaneously breathe at birth), the young woman is judged according to a standard that no one would ever ask of someone giving birth in a hospital to an expected baby. Whereas giving birth is ordinarily considered to be so painful that our culture doesn't think that women are in their right mind if they give birth without pain medication, these young women are expected to be skilled at newborn resuscitation and other obstetrical and midwifery skills immediately after giving birth unaided. I have read about these cases in the news media for thirty years. Most recently, a fourteen-year-old Houston girl gave birth at her friend's parents' apartment in April 2010, accompanied only by another fourteen-year-old and two eleven-year-olds. According to an officer who questioned the children, the baby was born alive but apparently suffocated because his head was covered with the amniotic sac. The young mother was charged with a felony charge of injury to a child.[14] Hopefully, the judge in this case will be merciful, but this has not always been the case in this country. We literally have no idea how many young women are serving long prison sentences in the US because they failed to resuscitate their babies and were charged with manslaughter or even murder. Trying to deal with this problem using the harsh punishments given these women does not serve as a deterrent. It only illustrates how much work we have to do to make it clear that women becoming mothers must have full human rights. We can and must change the culture of punishing mothers for not being perfect the moment that their babies emerge from their bodies. We need to not punish people for not knowing what we refused to teach them.

POSITIVE CHANGE IS POSSIBLE

I am convinced that it will be possible for women to agree on at least some of the changes that I have outlined in this book. I suggest that the goal of setting up a confidential system for accurate reporting and assessment of maternal deaths is one that all women, regardless of their politics, can agree upon. That is one important reason why I would like to see it rise to the top of a list of priorities for us to achieve. Most US women today have become used to feeling judged by each other—used to hearing endless polarizing arguments between mothers and women who have no children; those who stay in their homes with their children on a full-time basis and those who work outside the home; those who give birth with or without pain medication; those who favor home birth or hospital birth; those who breast-feed and those who bottle-feed; those who favor abortion rights and those who don't; and the list goes on and on. What a delicious thing it would be to take this issue that we could all agree on and make the solution happen. What a life-affirming and lifesaving campaign this would be. I'm sure that once we educate enough men about what is needed, they will pitch in and join our campaign for full human rights for mothers.

Using the social media to the greatest advantage, we should be able to bring about the needed changes in much less time than the seventy years it took for the suffragists to get the vote for women in the US. It didn't take very long at all for women to create the change needed to make it possible for their partners to be in the birth room with them; that happened almost overnight in hospitals in San Francisco and Palo Alto in the late sixties and then rapidly spread across the country. It doesn't have to take forever to get maternal deaths counted right, the postpartum needs of mothers recognized, the punishment regime modified to fit realities, and the positive role that midwives could play in birth fully utilized in the US. Let's make all these changes happen.

NOTES

1. Marsden Wagner, *Born in the USA: How a Broken Maternity System Must Be Fixed to Put Women and Children First* (Berkeley, CA: University of California Press, 2006).
2. Chris Woolston, "Medicine In a Small, Small Town," *AARP Bulletin*, June 1, 2010.
3. Charles Mahan, foreword to *Understanding the Dangers of Cesarean Birth: Making Informed Decisions, Nicette Jukelevics* (Westport, CT: Praeger, 2008).
4. Ibid.
5. Ibid.
6. Marsden Wagner, *Born in the USA: How a Broken Maternity System Must Be Fixed to Put Women and Children First* (Berkeley, CA: University of California Press, 2006).
7. Centers for Disease Control and Prevention, "Maternal mortality—United States, 1982-1996," *Morbidity and Mortality Weekly Report* 47, no. 34 (September 4, 1998): 705-707.
8. Hani K. Atrash, Sophie Alexander, and Cynthia Berg, "Maternal Mortality in Developed Countries: Not Just a Concern of the Past," *Obstetrics and Gynecology* 86, no. 4 (1995): 700-705.
9. Gwyneth Lewis, ed., and Confidential Enquiry into Maternal and Child Health, *Saving Mothers' Lives: Reviewing Maternal Deaths to Make Motherhood Safer—2003-2005* (London: CEMACH, 2007).
10. C. S. Landefeld, M. M. Chren, A. Myers, R. Geller, S. Robbins, and L. Goldman, "Diagnostic Yield of the Autopsy In a University Hospital and a Community Hospital," *New England Journal of Medicine* 318, no. 19 (1998): 1249-1254.
11. George D. Lundberg, "Low-Tech Autopsies In the Era of High-Tech Medicine: Continued Value for Quality Assurance and Patient Safety," *JAMA* 280, no. 14 (1998): 1273-1274.
12. John Golden, "Postnatal Problem Ruled to Be Cause of Soldier's Death," *Watertown Daily Times*, March 8, 2005.
13. See the "Virtual Quilt" at www.rememberthemothers.org.
14. Associated Press, "14-year-old Arrested After Her Newborn Suffocates," June 22, 2010.

Michaela at the Northern New Mexico Birth Center

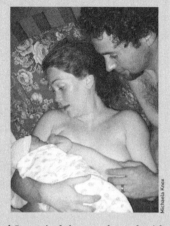

At 3:00 AM I realized I was in labor and we decided to start the drive to Taos right away. We suspected I would have a long labor, and we wanted the drive from Santa Fe to be relaxed. I had a bunch of mild contractions on the drive through the mountains. I was so excited! After nine months of waiting the time had come.

We spent the morning strolling around the plaza. We had French toast and window-shopped and I stopped for contractions whenever I needed to. It was the most thrilling morning of my life.

After lunch my water broke and everything shifted into high gear. My contractions consumed me completely. As I walked into the Birth Center I stopped for two contractions on the way. The midwife watched my face as I moved towards the pink room. She could tell that things had progressed. She gave us a huge smile. "That's what we like to see," she said. I immediately felt safe.

The midwives showed my husband Shawn how to press on my back during each contraction to counter some of the pressure. It helped tremendously. When I felt one coming, I would nod and he would get in position and press. As a little girl I remember watching ballerinas doing amazing things with their partners behind them supporting their every move. That's what this felt like. Shawn was my pillar and I was doing an amazing thing.

Throughout my labor I started chanting, "I can do it," whenever things started feeling really difficult. The midwives chimed in saying, "You *can* do it, you *are* doing it." I was surrounded with love and encouragement.

At one point someone handed me a mirror so I could take a look at how things were progressing. To me, my body looked no different. I started to panic. "Uh ... I don't see how this is going to work," I stammered to the apprentice. She looked me right in the eye and said, "Your body is about to teach something to your mind." The wisdom and certainty in her tone made me believe her. I finally let go of my mind and let my body take over.

My body knew that I had to move toward the pain to push my baby out. My mind couldn't suffer each contraction because my body was harnessing strength with each wave to bring my daughter into the world. Moments passed. I opened my eyes, and she was there. It was magic.

Giving birth was the most empowering moment of my life ... People told me it would hurt, people told me it would be hard, but no one told me that I would leave feeling like a superhero. That part was a surprise.

I have heard that a wave of amnesia falls over new mothers to make us forget the trials of childbirth, so that we will continue to procreate. I don't believe it. I think we remember every moment of the vomiting, the back pain, and the contractions that make our whole body scream. Remembering it all, we look into our babies' eyes and like heroes we move toward pregnancy once again, because we know that the light at the end of the tunnel is indescribable bliss.

—Michaela Knox

CHAPTER 9

The Kind of Obstetrics I Miss, and Its Great Defenders

In 1972, a wise Japanese obstetrician named Takao Kobayashi wrote:

> If you think carefully, the use of cesarean section, even as the last resort, has the potential to deconstruct delivery/obstetrics and to bring it closer to surgery. Thus there is a big contradiction inherent in obstetrics that the more you carry out cesarean sections, the greater the tendency that obstetrics will move toward surgery. So future obstetrics should be careful not to move toward cesarean section. We should recognize the true nature of such a move.[1]

Obstetrics in most every urbanized culture in the world have failed to heed this warning, to our detriment. I would like to take some time here to acknowledge those exceptional obstetricians who have risked their own careers to defend safe and mother-friendly care. These doctors deserve our praise, and our attention, as they can help to lead the way toward a more humane maternity care system around the world.

It has come to a point in the US where an obstetrician who maintains the 10-15 percent C-section rate that is within the range recommended by the World Health Organization may risk persecution. Dr. Colleen Murphy, an obstetrician-gynecologist from

Anchorage, Alaska, discovered this in 2005 when she found herself under investigation by the Alaska State Medical Board for what was called "an immediate risk to patients' health and safety." The supposedly risky behavior that caused the board to suspend both her license to practice obstetrics and her license to practice gynecology was her willingness to allow women who had had previous C-sections to try to give birth vaginally. So many women were able to achieve this goal that Dr. Murphy's C-section rate was reported to be 8 percent. She had to sit and listen to two and a half days of testimony from the state's witnesses about how dangerous she was to women and babies before she had an opportunity to defend herself. Once she was able to speak, she pointed out that she had always been careful to stay within the accepted guidelines for care in all her cases, and that too often doctors were choosing C-sections simply because they are more convenient and more profitable.

"You get about $700 more than the vaginal birth," she told the judge. "So you actually get paid more to do the quickest, easiest thing, compared to sitting at the bedside or being in the hospital with the patient."[2] This particular case of harassment ended happily for Dr. Murphy when Judge Hemenway reinstated her license after it had been suspended for two months. Yet, the prolonged incident made it clear that some doctors did not want Dr. Murphy's practice to inform women that giving birth vaginally after a previous C-section was possible and safe. At the same time, it is clear from some of the message boards that were active for at least two years after Dr. Murphy's reinstatement that Anchorage women who wanted a chance to have a vaginal birth after a C-section were still having trouble finding a doctor who would be supportive of this perfectly reasonable request.

What a bizarre situation! It's hard to think of a profession other than obstetrics in which members must risk being punished in order to maintain a high standard of practice with a full set of professional skills once considered essential for competent practice.

There is an unfortunate history of such nonsense, of course. In 1986, my friend Dr. Wendy Savage of London, England, was subjected to a similar witch hunt and suspended from medical practice for alleged incompetence in the management of five cases. Instead of submitting to a court or review board, Dr. Savage created an enormous upheaval when she demanded and received a public hearing of her case. She was reinstated when the allegations were not upheld and ultimately retired in 2000. Her book *Birth and Power* is a powerful account of her fight to restore her reputation and career after a ferocious attempt to force her out of practice for being conscientious about providing a kind of care that respected the needs of her patients.[3] Her rates of C-section and induction remained comparatively low, as both were rising sharply in the UK.

Another friend of mine, the late Dr. John Stevenson, a family physician from Victoria, Australia, ran into even worse trouble from fellow doctors—never from former patients, who continued to give him their support—when he began attending home births, helped by midwives whom he trained. He, too, raised the bar for his contemporaries by demonstrating that midwives backed by a competent and compassionate physician like himself could help almost every woman achieve a vaginal birth without high rates of medical intervention. The total C-section rate for more than 1,100 births over a period of eight years was 1.6 percent, which happened to be almost identical to the C-section rate that we midwives at The Farm achieved during approximately the same period. However, instead of being praised for this work, he was deregistered by the Medical Board of Victoria in 1984, and his medical career was finished. Even so, he continued to speak and teach midwifery, based upon the excellent outcomes of his years as a home birth practitioner. Dr. Stevenson's expertise is still recognized by midwives in the many countries where his reputation is known. He died at the age of eighty-nine, as I was finishing this book.

I was fascinated when Dr. Stevenson told me that before he

attended that first home birth, he would never have thought of doing such a thing; it was a pregnant woman who suffered from agoraphobia and was terrified of going to a hospital to give birth who managed to persuade him to assist her at home. That birth amazed him, as it taught him how much safer and easier birth could be when a woman gives birth in her own familiar surroundings ("With the mother in control, with her family present, with helpers of her own choosing, and with her baby given unrestricted love and welcoming," in his words) than when she is subjected to hospital routines. As I'll explain below, he has not been the only doctor to make such an observation.

Dr. Alfred Rockenschaub of Vienna, Austria, had results similar to those Dr. Stevenson and the midwives working with him did, but because the 44,500 births that took place under his care (working with midwives, of course) occurred in the large, well-known Ignaz Semmelweis Frauenklinik of which he was director between 1965 and 1985, his right to practice was never threatened.[4] Dr. Rockenschaub, who was also a professor at the midwifery school in Vienna, had some influence over midwifery education, but has yet to receive respect from members of his own profession. As I write, Dr. Rockenschaub spends some of his time trying to defend expert Austrian midwives who one by one come under fire for assisting at home births. When a baby dies during or after a hospital birth, that death is overlooked. No one will be punished. If, however, a baby died whose mother labored for any time at home, it will often be the case that the midwife or doctor or even the parents will be punished— as if their choice caused the death, regardless of what happened.

Dr. Tadashi Yoshimura, of Nagoya, Japan, is another obstetrician-gynecologist who took the less-trod path in obstetrics by tailoring his style of care according to the real needs of women and babies. According to Dr. Yoshimura, he began as a rather arrogant young man who was in favor of cutting-edge equipment and the latest medical practice (whatever that might be), the "flippant young manager

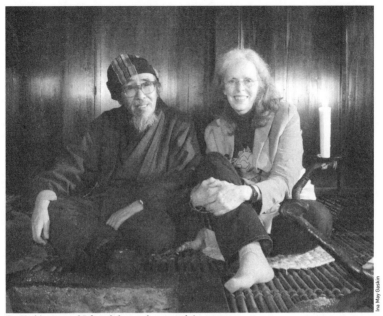

Dr. Yoshimura and I found that we have much in common.

of his obstetrician father's clinic," who loved to drive around in his Porsche. What changed him was the chance he had to observe how laboring women reacted to different styles of care. Having established a monitoring system in the clinic, he remembered looking into a monitor and being astonished to see the expression on the face of a young woman in labor who had become frightened after being left alone in the delivery room attached with cords to several poles. At the same time that he began to question much of what he had learned in medical school, he noticed a "mystic beauty" that women who were not frightened often exhibited during labor.[5] I know exactly what he means, because I have seen this too. In fact, I learned that when the mother is in this "beauty zone," complications are rare, and babies are born clean, rarely having any blood on them. Is this hard to believe? I acknowledge that it is, but it is, nevertheless, true.

Dr. Yoshimura now works with a staff of midwives and some younger obstetricians at his clinic, where thirty to forty babies are born each month. For one recent three-year period, the C-section rate was 3.2 percent, the forceps rate was 0 percent, and the rate of vacuum extraction was 0.5 percent. Is Dr. Yoshimura considered a national treasure? (Japan is one of those countries that does recognize its masters of certain arts.) Answer: not yet. But if Japan would take my advice, he would be given this recognition. It takes admirable courage for an obstetrician to break away from the herd mentality and respect the ability of women to give birth as their ancestors did. There are some professions that still recognize excellence within their own ranks and elevate those who demonstrate mastery to be teachers of those entering the profession. How good it would be if obstetrics joined their ranks.

In Hungary, my friend Dr. Ágnes Geréb, an obstetrician who has been part of Hungary's home birth movement for nearly two decades, has experienced an even greater wall of resistance than Dr. Stevenson did. When I began writing this chapter, Dr. Geréb was in prison on a twenty-three hour per day lock down. International pressure was necessary to spur her release to house arrest, but she still faces a five-year sentence, as of this writing. She is honored and respected by the families for whom she cared over the years. Her arrest took place a week before I arrived in Hungary to lecture in the fall of 2010, and I was hoping to meet her again. According to a report in the online journal *Budapest Moms* on October 6, 2010, the initial reason given for her arrest by four armed policeman was "suspicion of reckless endangerment committed during the line of duty." There was no precipitating event in which anyone came to harm. In fact, Dr. Geréb was televised being taken away from her home in chains a few hours after having called an ambulance for a pregnant woman who went into sudden labor during a consultation visit at her clinic; Dr. Geréb had just told the woman that her blood-clotting disorder would exclude her from giving birth there. At any rate, the baby, who was born at a hospital, survived and is healthy. But none of these facts kept her out of prison.

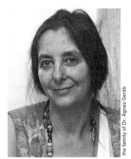

Dr. Ágnes Geréb.

Home birth is not illegal in Hungary. It is merely unregulated. For more than two decades, advocates for parents' choices to include home births and birthing centers have pressured Hungary's government to create a legal framework for birth choice, but to date, no laws or rules have been promulgated. Several public rallies were held in support of Dr. Geréb. In December 2010, the European Court of Human Rights heard the Ágnes Geréb case and criticized the "permanent threat" to health professionals in Hungary, emphasizing that, since Hungary is a member of the European Union, Hungarian womens' right to choose where to give birth is protected under Article 8 of the European Convention (right to private and

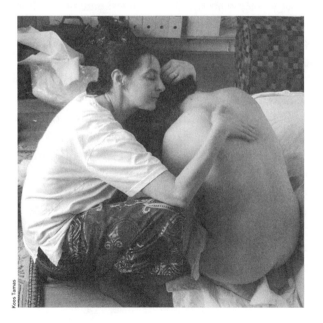

family life). The Hungarian Department of Health issues a promise to build birth centers and issue regulations for out-of-hospital births on December 20, 2010, Geréb's birthday. The following day, she was released to house arrest.

On October 7, 2010—a day after Dr. Geréb's arrest—one of her supporters explained why she planned to attend a public rally in an article titled "Home Birth in Hungary—One Apprentice Midwife's Experience," also published on *Budapest Moms*: "[T]his cause is bigger than just [Dr. Geréb, who] has courageously taken on the public fight, has accepted the role of martyr for the cause. And the Hungarian government is in serious remission for not having created the legal framework that would allow women to safely choose the location of their births and for professionals to legally attend to women who choose home births. That is just not right."

Dr. Geréb knows as well as I do that in any society, there are plural modes of birth. Even in societies that strongly discourage giving birth outside of hospitals, there will always be at least small numbers of women who will give birth at home or in other places, whether intentionally or not. I agree with the Japanese anthropologist Etsuko Matsuoka, who has provided a lucid explanation of how societies can benefit from taking tolerant stands regarding this situation. First, she says, out-of-hospital care (her discussion concerned Japanese maternity homes) serves as a breakwater to prevent childbirth from becoming too medicalized. Second, the midwifery practices that belong to these out-of-hospital care centers are considered by most midwives to represent the way midwifery *should* be: a source where the midwifery model of care prevails and can be pursued. During my visit to Tokyo in early 2010, I met many young midwifery students who yearned to have apprenticeships at a maternity home, because they found that their solely hospital-based training had filled them with fear about birth because of the overuse of medical technology that they were seeing there. Literally, every midwifery student whom I spoke with felt that she needed ways to develop confidence in women's ability to give birth. Maternity homes serve as sanctuaries of normal birth, which can help student midwives to develop a balanced image of midwifery practice. There need to be more of them—not fewer—if midwifery and obstetrics are to survive.

I have known too many doctors in the US who have had to be nimble to keep from getting in trouble for being too good at their work. These are the doctors who know that "saving a woman from labor pain" is not necessarily the biggest favor a doctor can do for every woman who is about to become a mother. There is a larger responsibility that also belongs to obstetrics (and midwifery) of teaching women not to fear the processes of their bodies. Whereas just a few decades ago women with breech presentations and multiples could count on giving birth without surgery, we now have the opposite situation—they are compelled to undergo surgery whether they like it or not. Obstetricians who dare to give women a chance to go into labor and experience an undisturbed birth may find themselves considered heretics by those who set the standards for the practice of obstetrics. The challenge is a big one, because there are now a lot of women who would agree with the woman who posted this on an online message board:

> I'm currently pregnant and I would vastly prefer a C-section to a vaginal delivery. I've done extensive research on the pros and cons of both and have come down strongly pro-C-section for myself. I'm aware of the risks, but the overall predictability of what the operation will entail and the ability to schedule the procedure tip it over the top for me.
>
> For every woman who wants to have a natural home birth in a bathtub in her living room there's a woman like me, who just wants the baby out safely with as little discomfort and as few messy bodily fluids as possible.

If for-profit hospitals are catering to that desire, I say check me in.

This woman is simultaneously under several illusions: (1) that she is fully aware of the true risks of elective C-sections; (2) that she will experience little discomfort having a C-section; (3) that there will be few "messy bodily fluids" involved in a surgical birth; and (4) that for-profit hospitals and her true interests are congruent. This mindset is spreading rapidly over the planet and is one of the factors that threaten to wipe out two essential professions—midwifery and obstetrics—and to replace them with surgery.

It is time to stop the witch hunt and save both midwifery and obstetrics by educating women, future midwives, and future doctors in the wisdom of nature's design for birth. All the women and men—midwives, nurses, obstetricians, and doulas—who preserve the midwifery model of care, and honor the medical oath to first do no harm, deserve our admiration and our support should they come under siege. Part of our work in reinvigorating the women's health movement must include creating communities and support networks, so that caretakers are enabled to do the right thing.

NOTES

1. Quoted in *Birth Models That Work*, edited by Robbie E. Davis-Floyd, Lesley Barclay, Betty-Anne Daviss, and Jan Tritten (Berkeley: University of California Press, 2009), 219.
2. http://www.mothering.com/discussions/archive/index.php/t-316940.html.
3. Wendy Savage, *Birth and Power, A Savage Enquiry Revisited: An Examination of Who Controls Childbirth and Who Controls Doctors* (London: Middlesex University Press, 2007).
4. Alfred Rockenschaub, *Gebären Ohne Aberglaube* (Vienna: Facultas Universitätsverlag, 2001).
5. Personal communication with Tadashi Yoshimura, November 1, 2010.

The Mother-Friendly Childbirth Initiative

THE FIRST CONSENSUS INITIATIVE OF THE COALITION FOR IMPROVING MATERNITY SERVICES (CIMS)

MISSION, PREAMBLE, AND PRINCIPLES

Mission

The Coalition for Improving Maternity Services (CIMS) is a coalition of individual and national organizations with concern for the care and well-being of mothers, babies, and families. Our mission is to promote a wellness model of maternity care that will improve birth outcomes and substantially reduce costs. This evidence-based mother-friendly, baby-friendly, and family-friendly model focuses on prevention and wellness as alternatives to high-cost screening, diagnosis, and treatment programs.

Preamble

Whereas

- In spite of spending far more money per capita on maternity and newborn care than any other country, the United States falls behind most industrialized countries in perinatal morbidity and mortality, and maternal mortality is four times greater for African-American women than for Euro-American women;
- Midwives attend the vast majority of births in those industrialized countries with the best perinatal outcomes, yet in the United

States, midwives are the principal attendants at only a small percentage of births;

- Current maternity and newborn practices that contribute to high costs and inferior outcomes include the inappropriate application of technology and routine procedures that are not based on scientific evidence;
- Increased dependence on technology has diminished confidence in women's innate ability to give birth without intervention;
- The integrity of the mother-child relationship, which begins in pregnancy, is compromised by the obstetrical treatment of mother and baby as if they were separate units with conflicting needs;
- Although breast-feeding has been scientifically shown to provide optimum health, nutritional, and developmental benefits to newborns and their mothers, only a fraction of US mothers are fully breast-feeding their babies by the age of six weeks;
- The current maternity care system in the United States does not provide equal access to health care resources for women from disadvantaged population groups, women without insurance, and women whose insurance dictates caregivers or place of birth;
Therefore,

We, the undersigned members of CIMS, hereby resolve to define and promote mother-friendly maternity services in accordance with the following principles.

Principles

We believe the philosophical cornerstones of mother-friendly care to be as follows:

Normalcy of the Birth Process
- Birth is a normal, natural, and healthy process.
- Women and babies have the inherent wisdom necessary for birth.

- Babies are aware, sensitive human beings at the time of birth and should be acknowledged and treated as such.
- Breast-feeding provides the optimum nourishment for newborns and infants.
- Birth can safely take place in hospitals, birth centers, and homes.
- The midwifery model of care, which supports and protects the normal birth process, is the most appropriate for the majority of women during pregnancy and birth.

Empowerment

- A woman's confidence and ability to give birth and to care for her baby are enhanced or diminished by every person who gives her care and by the environment in which she gives birth.
- A mother and baby are distinct yet interdependent during pregnancy, birth, and infancy. Their interconnectedness is vital and must be respected.
- Pregnancy, birth, and the postpartum period are milestone events in the continuum of life. These experiences profoundly affect women, babies, fathers, and families and have important and long-lasting effects on society.

Autonomy

Every woman should have the opportunity to:
- Have a healthy and joyous birth experience for herself and her family, regardless of her age or circumstances;
- Give birth as she wishes in an environment in which she feels nurtured and secure, and her emotional well-being, privacy, and personal preferences are respected;
- Have access to the full range of options for pregnancy, birth, and care for her baby, and full access to accurate information on all available birthing sites, caregivers, and practices;
- Receive accurate and up-to-date information about the bene-

fits and risks of all procedures, drugs, and tests suggested for use during pregnancy, birth, and the postpartum period, with the rights to informed consent and informed refusal;

♦ Receive support for making informed choices about what is best for her and her baby based on her individual values and beliefs.

Do No Harm

♦ Interventions should not be applied routinely during pregnancy, birth, or the postpartum period. Many standard medical tests, procedures, technologies, and drugs carry risks to both mother and baby and should be avoided in the absence of specific indications for their use.

♦ If complications arise during pregnancy, birth, or the postpartum period, medical treatments should be evidence-based.

Responsibility

♦ Each caregiver is responsible for the quality of care she or he provides.

♦ Maternity care practice should be based not on the needs of the caregiver or provider but solely on the needs of the mother and child.

♦ Each hospital and birth center is responsible for the periodic review and evaluation, according to current scientific evidence, of the effectiveness, risks, and rates of use of its medical procedures for mothers and babies.

♦ Society, through both its government and the public health establishment, is responsible for ensuring access to maternity services for all women, and for monitoring the quality of those services.

♦ Individuals are ultimately responsible for making informed choices about the health care they and their babies receive.

These principles give rise to the following steps, which support, protect, and promote mother-friendly maternity services.

Ten Steps of the Mother-Friendly Childbirth Initiative for Mother-Friendly Hospitals, Birth Centers, and Home Birth Services

To receive CIMS designation as "mother-friendly," a hospital, birth center, or home birth service must carry out the above philosophical principles by fulfilling the Ten Steps of Mother-Friendly Care.

A mother-friendly hospital, birth center, or home birth service:

1. Offers all birthing mothers:

* Unrestricted access to the birth companions of her choice, including fathers, partners, children, family members, and friends;
* Unrestricted access to continuous emotional and physical support from a skilled woman—for example, a doula or labor-support professional;
* Access to professional midwifery care.

2. Provides accurate descriptive and statistical information to the public about its practices and procedures for birth care, including measures of interventions and outcomes.

3. Provides culturally competent care—that is, care that is sensitive and responsive to the specific beliefs, values, and customs of the mother's ethnicity and religion.

4. Provides the birthing woman with the freedom to walk, move about, and assume the positions of her choice during labor and birth (unless restriction is specifically required to correct a complication) and discourages the use of the lithotomy (flat on back with legs elevated) position.

5. Has clearly defined policies and procedures for:

- collaborating and consulting throughout the perinatal period with other maternity services, including communicating with the original caregiver when transfer from one birth site to another is necessary;
- linking the mother and baby to appropriate community resources, including prenatal and postdischarge follow-up and breast-feeding support.

6. Does not routinely employ practices and procedures that are unsupported by scientific evidence, including but not limited to the following:

- shaving
- enemas
- IVs (intravenous drip)
- withholding nourishment or water
- early rupture of membranes
- electronic fetal monitoring

Other interventions are limited as follows:
- Has an induction rate of 10 percent or less
- Has an episiotomy rate of 20 percent or less, with a goal of 5 percent or less
- Has a total cesarean rate of 10 percent or less in community hospitals and 15 percent or less in tertiary care (high-risk) hospitals
- Has a VBAC (vaginal birth after cesarean) rate of 60 percent or more, with a goal of 75 percent or more

7. Educates staff in nondrug methods of pain relief and does not promote the use of analgesic or anesthetic drugs not specifically required to correct a complication.

8. Encourages all mothers and families, including those with sick or premature newborns or infants with congenital problems, to touch, hold, breast-feed, and care for their babies to the extent compatible with their conditions.

9. Discourages nonreligious circumcision of the newborn.

10. Strives to achieve the WHO-UNICEF "Ten Steps of the Baby-Friendly Hospital Initiative" to promote successful breast-feeding:

1. Have a written breast-feeding policy that is routinely communicated to all health care staff
2. Train all health care staff in skills necessary to implement this policy
3. Inform all pregnant women about the benefits and management of breast-feeding
4. Help mothers initiate breast-feeding within a half hour of birth
5. Show mothers how to breast-feed and how to maintain lactation even if they should be separated from their infants
6. Give newborn infants no food or drink other than breast milk unless medically indicated
7. Practice "rooming in": allow mothers and infants to remain together twenty-four hours a day
8. Encourage breast-feeding on demand
9. Give no artificial teat or pacifiers (also called dummies or soothers) to breast-feeding infants
10. Foster the establishment of breast-feeding support groups and refer mothers to them on discharge from hospitals or clinics

List of Resources Pertinent to the Midwifery Model of Care

Pregnancy and Birth

Birthing the Future
PO Box 1040
Bayfield, CO 81122
(970) 884-4005
www.birthingthefuture.com

Coalition for Improving Maternity
   Services (CIMS)
The Mother-Friendly Childbirth Initiative
CIMS National Office
1500 Sunday Drive, Suite 102
Raleigh, NC 27607
(919) 863-9482
www.motherfriendly.org
info@motherfriendly.org

The Childbirth Connection
260 Madison Avenue, 8th floor
New York, NY 10016
(212) 777-5000
www.childbirthconnection.org

Group B Strep Association (GBSA)
PO Box 16515
Chapel Hill, NC 27516
www.groupbstrep.org

International Center for Traditional
   Childbearing
ICTC Midwives
PO Box 11923
Portland, OR 97211
(503) 460-9324
www.ictcmidwives.org

Postpartum Support International
6706 SW 54th Avenue
Portland, OR 97219
(800) 944-4PPD
www.postpartum.net

National Association of Postpartum
   Care Services
800 Detroit Street
Denver, CO 80206
(800) 45-DOULA
www.napcs.org

Doulas and Childbirth Education

Association of Labor Assistants and
   Childbirth Educators (ALACE)
12 Batchelder Street, Suite 2
Boston, MA 02125-2653
(877) 334-IBWP
www.alace.org

Birth Works International
PO Box 2045
Medford, NJ 08055
(888) 862-4784
www.birthworks.org

Birthing from Within
PO Box 60259
Santa Barbara, CA 93160
(805) 964-6611
www.birthingfromwithin.com

The Bradley Method of Natural
  Childbirth
PO Box 5224
Sherman Oaks, CA 91413
(800) 4-A BIRTH
www.bradleybirth.com

DONA International
1582 S. Parker Road, Suite 201
Denver, CO 80231
(888) 788-DONA
www.dona.org

HypnoBirthing Institute
PO Box 810
Epsom, NH 03234
www.hypnobirthing.com

International Childbirth Education
  Association (ICEA)
1500 Sunday Drive, Suite 102
Raleigh, NC 27607
(800) 624-4934
www.icea.org

Lamaze International
2025 M Street, NW, Suite 800
Washington DC 20036-3309
(800) 368-4404
www.lamaze.org

Midwifery

American College of Nurse-
  Midwifery (ACNM)
8403 Colesville Road, Suite 1550
Silver Spring, MD 20910
(240) 485-1800
www.midwife.org

Midwives Alliance of North America
  (MANA)
611 Pennsylvania Avenue, SE, Suite
  1700
Washington DC 20003
(888) 923-6262
www.mana.org

Further Reading/Films

BOOKS

Effective Birth Preparation: Your Practical Guide to a Better Birth
Maggie Howell, Founder of Natal Hypnotherapy
Intuition UN Ltd., ISBN 978-1-90522-059-5
www.natalhypnotherapy.co.uk

Mainstreaming Midwives: The Politics of Change
Edited by Robbie Davis-Floyd and Christine Barbara Johnson
Routledge, Taylor & Francis Group, ISBN 978-0-41593-151-9

Birth Models That Work
Edited by Robbie Davis-Floyd, Lesley Barclay, Betty-Anne Daviss, and Jan
    Tritten
University of California Press, ISBN 978-0-52025-891-4

*Born in the USA: How a Broken Maternity System Must Be Fixed to Put
    Women and Children First*
Marsden Wagner
University of California Press, ISBN 978-0-52025-633-0

*Pushed: The Painful Truth About Childbirth and Modern
    Maternity Care*
Jennifer Block
Da Capo Press, ISBN 978-0-73821-166-4

Birth: The Surprising History of How We Are Born
Tina Cassidy
Grove Press, ISBN 978-0-80214-324-2

Childbirth Without Fear: The Principles and Practice of Natural Childbirth
Grantly Dick-Read, with a Foreword by Michel Odent
Pinter & Martin Classics, ISBN 978-0-95309-646-6
www.pinterandmartin.com

Orgasmic Birth: Your Guide to a Safe, Satisfying, and Pleasurable Birth Experience
Elizabeth Davis and Debra Pascali-Bonaro
Rodale Books, ISBN 978-1-60529-528-2
www.orgasmicbirth.com

Gentle Birth, Gentle Mothering
Dr. Sarah J. Buckley
One Moon Press, ISBN 978-0-975807705
www.sarahjbuckley.com

*Your Best Birth: Know All Your Options, Discover the Natural Choices, and
	Take Back the Birth Experience*
Ricki Lake and Abby Epstein
Wellness Central, ISBN 978-0-446-53814-5

Birth and Power: A Savage Enquiry Revisited
Wendy Savage
Middlesex University Press, ISBN 978-1-904750-58-1

*How to Avoid an Unnecessary Caesarean: A Handbook for Women Who Want a
	Natural Birth*
Helen Churchill and Wendy Savage
Middlesex University Press, ISBN 978-1-904750-16-1

The Faceless Caesarean
Caroline Oblasser
Edition Riedenburg, Austria, ISBN 978-3-8370-7560-1

Lady's Hands, Lion's Heart
Carol Leonard
Bad Beaver Publishing, ISBN 978-0-615-19550-6

Granny Midwives and Black Women Writers: Double-Dutched Readings
Valerie Lee
Routledge, ISBN 978-0-415-91508-3

*Birth in Four Cultures: A Crosscultural Investigation of Childbirth in Yucatan,
	Holland, Sweden, and the United States*
Brigitte Jordan
Waveland Press, Fourth Edition, ISBN 978-0-88133-717-4

Childbirth Wisdom: From the World's Oldest Societies
Judith Goldsmith
Talman Co., ISBN 978-0-936184-10-4

Creating Your Birth Plan: The Definitive Guide to a Safe and Empowering Birth
Marsden Wagner and Stephanie Gunning
Perigee Trade, First Edition, ISBN 978-1-61554-339-7

VIDEOS

Laboring Under an Illusion: Mass Media Childbirth vs. The Real Thing
A Documentary by Vicki Elson

The Business of Being Born
Produced by Ricki Lake, Directed by Abby Epstein
Official Selection: 2007 Tribeca Film Festival
www.thebusinessofbeingborn.com

Orgasmic Birth: The Best-Kept Secret
Directed by Debra Pascali-Bonaro
www.orgasmicbirth.com

No Woman, No Cry
A Film by Christy Turlington Burns
www.everymothercounts.org

A Breech in the System: A Natural Breech Against All Odds
A Documentary by Karin Ecker
www.abreechinthesystem.com

Miss Margaret: The Story of an Alabama Granny Midwife
The Home Birth Series, Volume I
Sage Femme
PO Box 973
Tiburon, CA 94920
(415) 847-6252
www.sagefemme.com

Birth Day
The Home Birth Series, Volume II
Sage Femme
PO Box 973
Tiburon, CA 94920
(415) 847-6252
www.sagefemme.com

Home Birth: The Spirit, The Science, and The Mother
The Home Birth Series, Volume III, Part 1
Sage Femme
PO Box 973
Tiburon, CA 94920
(415) 847-6252
www.sagefemme.com

Working Women in Labor
In the Doula Spirit
Created by Working Women Productions
www.feliciaroche.com

Birthing: What Dads Can Do
Directed by Heather Bruce, an acupuncturist/naturopath/herbalist from Brisbane, Australia
www.heatherbrucebooks.com.au

Breast is Best
Directed by Gro Nylander, MD, PhD, Department of Obstetrics
A prize-winning DVD for midwives, lactation consultants, postpartum doulas, and others, used in more than fifty countries.
HEALTH INFO, Video Vital AS
PO Box 5058 Majorstua
0301 Oslo, Norway
HEALTH-INFO@videovital.no

Biological Nurturing: Laid-back Breastfeeding
Dr. Suzanne Colson
www.biologicalnurturing.com

What Babies Want: An Exploration of the Consciousness of Infants
A Documentary by Debby Takikawa and narrated by Noah Wyle
Beginnings Inc., a Resource Center for Children and Families
PO Box 681
Los Olivos, CA 93441
(800) 893-5070
www.whatbabieswant.com

The Happiest Baby on the Block
Dr. Harvey Karp
www.thehappiestbaby.com

The Farm Midwifery Center:
Preliminary Report of 2,844 Pregnancies, 1970–2010

Total accepted for care:	2,844	
Births completed at home	2,694	94.7%
Transports to hospital	148	5.2%
Cesareans	50	1.7%
First-time mothers	1,048	36.8%
Multiparas	1,796	63.2%
Grand multiparas	243	8.5%
Total Breech	99	3.5%
Frank	75	76%
Footling/kneeling	24	24%
C-section rate for breech		<10%
Twins	17 sets	
Vaginal births	17 sets	
Vaginal births after hospital transport	2 sets	
Postpartum hemorrhage	46	1.7%
Vaginal birth after cesarean	127	(123 managed to have vaginal births) 96.8% rate of success

Intact perineum	1,817	68.7%
1st degree tear	485	19.4%
2nd degree tear	87	3.2%
3rd degree tear	8	0.3%
4th degree tear	1	0.04%
Meconium staining	304	11.5%
Vacuum extraction	4	.04%
Forceps deliveries	10	0.37%
Brow presentations	10	
Vaginally born	5	
Face presentations	13	
Vaginally born	12	
Preeclampsia	11	0.4%
Maternal mortality	0	
Maternal morbidity	0	

Neonatal mortality

2000–2010	0 of 631 labors
1990–1999	1 of 372 labors
1980–1989	1 of 758 labors
1970–1979	2 of 1,083 labors

Neonatal mortality rate	1.7 deaths per 1,000 births

Every birth attended by our midwives—including those of Pamela's and my training period—is represented in this set of statistics.

Glossary

Accoucheur: man midwife.

Amniotic fluid: Fluid that is produced by and is inside the water bag during pregnancy.

Amniotic fluid embolism: A complication that is often fatal for the mother, in which amniotic fluid is pushed into the fetal circulation beneath an edge of the placenta. AFE is more likely in hard labors, or those that are augmented.

Amyotrophic lateral sclerosis (ALS): A disease that involves degeneration of the nerves within the brain and spinal cord that control motor activity.

Autoimmune disorders: Diseases in which the body's immune system mistakenly attacks healthy cells and tissues.

Blood-letting: A common medical practice that continued throughout the 19th century that involved cutting the vein to remove supposedly "excess" blood.

Catecholamines: A family of hormones that are released by the body in response to fear, hunger, and cold. These are the "fight-or-flight," or stress, hormones.

Cytotec: Misoprostol is the generic name of this drug, which was approved by the FDA for ulcer prevention, but not for use in labor. Often used as a "cervical ripener," or for induction, it can cause uterine rupture, amniotic fluid embolism, severe birth injury, or death to mother or baby.

Dermatomyositis: A rare type of inflammation of the muscles and skin that has been linked to silicone exposure.

DES daughters: Daughters of women of the estimated 1.5 million women who took diethylstilbestrol (DES) under the mistaken notion that this would prevent miscarriages. Nine out of every ten DES daughters had deformed reproductive systems.

Diethylstilbestrol (DES): A synthetic estrogen that was developed in 1938. DES was prescribed by doctors for women who experienced miscarriages or premature deliveries. Since 1971, DES has been linked to an increased risk of clear cell carcinoma of the vagina and cervix, infertility, and pregnancy complications in women exposed to DES before birth (in the womb).

Doula: Labor companion.

Fibromyalgia: A syndrome of symptoms that includes muscle and joint pain, stiffness, and relentless fatigue that occurs mostly in women of childbearing age.

Hypertension: High blood pressure.

Lever: Forceps.

Multiple sclerosis (MS): A progressive disease of the central nervous system.

Palpation: The art of assessing fetal size and position with the hands applied to the woman's abdomen.

Placenta increta: When the placenta attaches itself to the uterine muscle and cannot be released in the normal way after the birth of the baby. More common in a scarred uterus.

Pseudocyesis: False pregnancy.

Puerperal fever: Infection of the uterus following birth.

Pulmonary embolism: A deep vein thrombosis that dislodges and goes to the lungs. It is often fatal.

Rheumatoid arthritis: A severe arthritic disorder involving inflammation of the joints.

Scleroderma: A thickening of fiber in skin and tissue surrounding the vital organs.

Systemic lupus erythematosus: Inflammation of connective tissue, joints, and kidneys. The disease tends to run in families and is more common in women than in men.

Teratogenic: Poisonous to the embryo or fetus.

Acknowledgments

I owe Crystal Yakacki a huge debt of gratitude for persuading me to write this book. Her gentle insistence that I delve into areas of women's health that have great importance to women of her generation pushed me into widening my scope of what women today need to know about their bodies and the products and services that are being marketed directly to them.

I want to thank Ani DiFranco, Heidi Knoop, Charlotte Hamilton, Chloe Labouerie, Teresa Bissen, Keri, Skylar Browning, and Michaela Knox for sharing their stories with me.

Amnesty International USA deserves my gratitude for greatly increasing the visibility of the Safe Motherhood Quilt Project and for applying the language of human rights to the important area of women's choices in childbirth.

Dr. Frank Vasey gets a big thank you from me for carrying on his lonely but vital quest to bring awareness to the connection between breast implants and various autoimmune disorders.

My thanks go to Saraswathi Vedam, CNM, for sharing her and her colleagues' important critique of the Wax study.

Last but not least, I thank Drs. Charles Mahan and Marsden Wagner for devoting so much of their time and energy to educating women and caregivers about what maternity care should be.

Index

natural birth on, 20–27
See also birth centers; birth stories
on The Farm; Gaskin, Ina May
fathers
and birth process, 167–168, 171–173
personal story, 173–178
role after birth, 178–179
fear of birth, 27–29, 54, 59–61, 78–79
as abnormal, 36, 60
and technology, 4, 14
See also Hodge, Dr. Hugh L.; medical men; pain in childbirth
feminism
and abortion, 18–19
and birth, 19
second-wave feminism, 17–19, 69
women-centered ethic, 41–42
and women's' health care, 143–146
See also de Beauvoir, Simone; empowerment; motherhood; second-wave feminism; women-centered ethic
forceps, 59, 64, 77–78
percent of deliveries with, 21, 61
See also medicalization of birth

G
___

Gaskin, Ina May
career as midwife, 21–27
Gaskin maneuver, 195
surgery performed on, 21, 24
See also The Farm Midwifery Center
Geréb, Dr. Ágnes, 217–218
See also human rights

H
___

Hodge, Dr. Hugh L.
and fear of birth, 59, 79
midwives as competitors, 74, 87
and scare tactics, 74
See also medical men
home births, 72, 89–90
importance of surroundings, 39, 214
loss of rights, 90
postpartum care, 203–205
problematic studies on, 91–98
See also Dutch care system; Teresa at Home
hormones
adrenaline, 25, 30, 33, 171
beta-endorphins, 34–35, 40, 53
oxytocin, 33–34, 40, 53, 170–171
role of in birth, 25, 33–37, 40, 52–53
See also pain in childbirth
hospitals, 81, 75, 114, 200
humanized birth principles, 9
human rights
Deadly Delivery: The Maternal Health Care Crisis in the USA (Amnesty International), 129, 131
and birth, 7, 217, 220
women-centered ethic, 41–42
and women's maternity care, 6,191–194, 207, 217
See also Geréb, Dr. Ágnes; maternal mortality rate

ABOUT THE AUTHOR

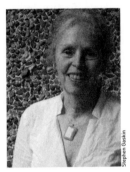

Stephen Gaskin

Called "the midwife of modern midwifery" by *Salon*, INA MAY GASKIN has practiced for nearly forty years at the internationally lauded Farm Midwifery Center. She is the only midwife for whom an obstetric maneuver has been named (Gaskin maneuver). She is the author of *Spiritual Midwifery, Ina May's Guide to Childbirth*, and *Ina May's Guide to Breastfeeding.*

ABOUT SEVEN STORIES PRESS

SEVEN STORIES PRESS is an independent book publisher based in New York City, with distribution throughout the world. We publish works of the imagination by such writers as Nelson Algren, Russell Banks, Octavia E. Butler, Ani DiFranco, Assia Djebar, Ariel Dorfman, Coco Fusco, Barry Gifford, Hwang Sok-yong, Peter Plate, Lee Stringer, and Kurt Vonnegut, to name a few, together with political titles by voices of conscience, including the Boston Women's Health Collective, Noam Chomsky, Angela Y. Davis, Human Rights Watch, Derrick Jensen, Ralph Nader, Loretta Napoleoni, Gary Null, Project Censored, Ted Rall, Barbara Seaman, Alice Walker, Gary Webb, and Howard Zinn, among many others. Seven Stories Press believes publishers have a special responsibility to defend free speech and human rights, and to celebrate the gifts of the human imagination, wherever we can. For additional information, visit www.sevenstories.com.